Genetics and Ageing

Interdisciplinary Topics in Gerontology

Vol. 14

Series Editor
H.P. von Hahn, Basel

S. Karger · Basel · München · Paris · London · New York · Sydney

Genetics and Ageing

F.A. Lints

Laboratoire de Génétique, Université Catholique de Louvain, Louvain-La-Neuve, Belgique

27 figures and 19 tables, 1978

S. Karger · Basel · München · Paris · London · New York · Sydney

Interdisciplinary Topics in Gerontology

Vol. 9: Cellular Ageing: Concepts and Mechanisms, Part I: General Concepts. Mechanisms I.: Fidelity of Information Flow. Editor: *R.G. Cutler* (Richardson, Tex.).
VI + 218 p., 13 fig., 10 tab., 1976. ISBN 3–8055–2283–5

Vol. 10: Cellular Ageing: Concepts and Mechanisms, Part II: Mechanisms II: Translation, Transcription and Structural Properties. Editor: *R.G. Cutler* (Richardson, Tex.).
VI + 130 p., 10 fig., 35 tab., 1976. ISBN 3–8055–2284–3

Vol. 11: Multidisciplinary Gerontology: A Structure for Research in Gerontology in a Developed Country. Editor: *I.R. Mackay* (Melbourne).
VI + 118 p., 23 fig., 17 tab., 1977. ISBN 3–8055–2679–2

Vol. 12: Lens Ageing and Development of Senile Cataracts. Workshop on Ageing of the Lens, held after the 18th Meeting of the Association for Eye Research, Bonn 1977. Editor: *O. Hockwin* (Bonn).
XII + 296 p., 170 fig., 47 tab., 1978. ISBN 3–8055–2876–0

Vol. 13: Gerontological Aspects of Eye Research. Selected papers of the 18th Meeting of the Association for Eye Research, Bonn 1977. Editor: *O. Hockwin* (Bonn).
XII + 260 p., 165 fig., 53 tab., 1978. ISBN 3–8055–2877–9

National Library of Medicine Cataloging in Publication
    Lints, F.A.
    Genetics and ageing / F.A. Lints. – –
    Basel ; New York : Karger 1978.
    (Interdisciplinary topics in gerontology ; v. 14)
    1. Aging 2. Genetics I. Title II. Series
    W1 IN679 v.14 WT 104.3 L761g
    ISBN 3–8055–2891–4

Contents

Contents

Acknowledgments

I wish to express my gratitude to my co-workers and, first of all, to *C.V. Lints*, without whose help this small book would probably never have been done; many thanks are also due to my other co-workers, past and present: *G. Gruwez, C. Hoste, M.H. Soliman* and *J. Stoll*.

I am particularly indebted to my colleagues *J. Beardmore, D. Gershon, A. Macieira-Coelho* and *H.P. von Hahn* who were kind enough to read the entirety or parts of the manuscript and whose criticisms unquestionably contributed to my work. Shortcomings which remain are, of course, my responsibility.

In addition, I am grateful to the many colleagues who granted me the permission to reproduce their photographs or illustrations: *E. Ashby, A.N. Bozcuk, G.E. Bradford, H.J. Curtis, C.W. Daniel, J. Delcour, J. Eklund, A. Elens, R. Holliday, J.L. Jinks, A.I. Lansing, A. Macieira-Coelho, G.M. Martin, K. Mather, J. Maynard Smith, O. Mühlbock, M.H. Ross, J. Smith-Sonneborn, T.M. Sonneborn, F. Vogel.*

Plus ne suis ce que j'ai été,
Et plus ne saurais jamais l'être.

Clement Marot (1495–1544)

Le tems s'en va, le tems s'en va, ma Dame
Las! le tems non, mais nous nous en allons.

Pierre de Ronsard (1524–1585)

Foreword

In the mind of the 'man in the street', ageing and longevity have always been linked to the idea of inheritance. The familial heritability of a long individual life-span is generally considered a well-proven fact and above any reasonable doubt ('If you want to live long, choose long-lived parents'). And yet, as Prof. *Lints* vividly demonstrates in the present volume, the causal relationship between genetic factors, on the one hand, and phenotypic ageing processes at the level of the physiology of the individual, on the other hand, is an exceedingly complex one and does not yield readily to simple analysis. This may be one reason why, as I believe, this very fundamental aspect of the ageing problem has so far not been sufficiently taken into account in much of experimental gerontological research.

Much of the material presented and discussed here comes from studies of short-lived invertebrates, the ideal organisms for genetic studies. The author himself has contributed pioneering studies on ageing mechanisms in *Drosophila*, and a *Bibliography on Longevity, Ageing and Parental Age Effects* in this organism (*Gerontology 22*: 380–410, 1976). It is much to his credit that here he ventures far outside his personal specialty and tackles the difficult and still poorly explored field of genetic ageing factors in vertebrates, and particularly in mammals and man. Recently, the concept of a species-specific, and therefore genetically determined maximum life-span potential has become a focus of discussion in gerontology, and Prof. *Lints* enters the forum with a clear and pointed analysis of the available evidence, sorting out the grains of hard fact from the chaff of speculations.

This is the kind of critical writing that experimental gerontology needs. It is truly interdisciplinary and will appeal equally to geneticists and gerontologists. The problem of genetic regulation of life-span and ageing is still a most controversial one, and I am certain that the present volume will stimulate others to enter this fascinating field of study.

H.P. von Hahn

I. Introduction

The juxtaposition of the words 'genetics' and 'ageing' may sound strange to the ears of a geneticist. One should say − *must* sound strange. Indeed, a rapid survey of a dozen or so of recent textbooks of genetics shows that, without exception, the authors judge that a few lines, half a page or so, are enough to report on the relations between age and genetics.

For a gerontologist, the words genetics and ageing may perhaps also look strange. It should appear from this assay that the geneticist's approach, who tries to understand, say terata or a biosynthetic pathway by searching for, or even by provoking, mutations still remains unfamiliar to the gerontologist. Indeed, gerontological studies remain mostly confined to a phenomenological approach of the variation which accompanies the passage of time in the living being.

The relations between genetics and ageing may be examined from two different points of view. The first series of questions bears to the amount and type of genetic control in the phenomenon of ageing and death. We will not review or discuss the whole of the theories of ageing which have been proposed and advocated in the last 30 years. This has been done (see, for instance, *Theoretical Aspects of Aging* edited by *Rockstein,* 1974a). Furthermore, with *von Hahn* (1973), we feel that most, if not all, theories of ageing may be reassembled in two groups. In the first group, ageing and death are considered to be more or less random events; in this category fall the mutation and derived theories of ageing as, for instance, the famous error-catastrophe theory of ageing. The theoreticians of the second group assume that ageing and death are non-random events. They consider both these phenomena as being linked to growth and development, as being programmed by a series of coordinated information.

On that account the meaning of programme and of information should be specified. Programmation should not be considered as synonymous to preformation or predetermination. Embryogenesis, morphogenesis, growth, development are the result of cellular activities, i.e. of interactions between genetic information and intracellular, extracellular or even extraorganismic elements. The programme constitutes a scheme of activities, probably fixed in a part of the genome, i.e. in the genetical information in the narrow sense of the word; intracellular, extracellular, extraorganismic elements are provided, of course, by the environment, but also by genetical information in the large sense of the word. Genetical information, in the wide sense of the word, is not uniquely constituted of information specified by genes, in the Mendelian sense of the word, but also by cytoplasmic elements, cortical properties, the molecular geography of the cells, including the fertilized egg, all of which may influence to a considerable extent the spatio-temporal fate of a developing organism. To make a comparison, the final result delivered by a computer depends both on an invariable programme and on a variable set of data provided to the machine.

A second series of questions pertaining to genetics and ageing relates to the possible importance of parental age on the faithful transmission of information from parent to offspring. What kind of phenotypic variation in offspring can be correlated with variation in parental age? In how far is this variation transmissible? What is it due to? Is it caused by programmed, or by chance, modifications in the genetic information or in some other type of information? Is there any relation between those modifications and ageing itself? These are the questions which need to be answered.

To support a non-random theory of ageing, the phenomenon being considered as programmed, as linked to growth and development, does not mean that we believe to have reached the ideal of a gerontologist. There was a time where the purpose of gerontologists was to develop a universal theory of ageing which would apply perfectly to all forms of life. Few, I believe, actually think that such a purpose is attainable, at least in the near future. There are too many forms of life and too many evolutionary strategies of life. The mayfly plays its part in less than 24 h; the Galapagos' tortoise needs more than a century to do the same thing. They both appear perfectly well adapted, they both fit perfectly in their ecological niche. For the time being, to sketch a frame within which the chain of reasoning may be carried on appears to be a sufficient aim.

II. Genetics and the Control of Ageing and Death

As everyone knows, genetics is the science of heredity and variation. Heredity is that process which brings about the similarity between parents and progeny. Variation is the occurrence of differences among individuals of a population or among populations. Variation may be due either to mutations or to the environment.

In the present study of ageing and death, our first and foremost interest will be for what may be called 'normal' ageing and death. The signification of 'normal' ageing and death is known to everybody, though it can hardly be precisely defined. This is a familiar although undefinable notion just as the concepts of species or of life. Gross variations in ageing and death due to major genetic mutations — Werner's syndrome or progeria, for instance — are of no direct relevance to our problem. In the same way, large environmental disturbances due, for instance, to infections, diseases, accidents, ill-balanced or insufficient nutrition, are not directly relevant. This does not mean that these two types of variation are to be neglected. They may in some aspects and to a certain extent mimic what normal ageing is.

The hereditary basis of ageing and death seems to be generally accepted by most authors. This is, however, not very obvious from the few experimental results. In contrast with that general agreement, the fact that for the last decades the causes of death have not been searched at the level of genetic mechanisms appears as a paradox. In fact, most theoreticians and experimentalists alike, did look for a mechanism the release of which would be purely random. The publication of a great number of works induced by recent claims concerning the error-catastrophe theory of ageing, a modern version of the older mutation theory, is a sufficient argument to demonstrate that point. It is because of that great number of publications that a chapter will be devoted to the random theory in order to verify its validity.

In contrast, very few experiments have been designed to test the idea of ageing, natural, orderly, strict phenomenon, extension of development and maturity, announcer of death. This is all the more strange that no biologist will dispute the developmental nature of the successive stages of life from birth to maturity, through infancy, childhood, adolescence. When one comes to senescence, which culminates in death, one ignores, or prefers to ignore, that it is a normal part of a total process. But where does maturity stop and where does senescence start?

There was a time where developmental changes were considered as due to permanent genetic changes in the genetic material of the somatic cells. Today, nobody would advocate such a view for a lot of reasons that are known to everybody. The permanent genetic change interpretation of senescence and death persisted for a longer time and, I guess, still persists through its modernized version of the error-catastrophe theory. One may wonder to what extent the horror of death, that apparently perfect nonsense event, conditions the theories of ageing. Thus, from a typical human, i.e. a so-called reasonable point of view, it is inadmissible to account for that unreasonable event in terms of a sequential, orderly and admirable process. It becomes reasonably admissible only in terms of accidents, indeterminacy, disaster, tragedy or catastrophe.

A. The Hereditary Basis of Ageing

According to many authorities, there is apparently ample and classical evidence that ageing and death are tô some extent genetically controlled. A number of review papers dealing with the topic have been published (*Glass,* 1943, 1960; *Clark,* 1964; *Comfort,* 1964; *Rockstein,* 1974b). These authors would claim that the strongest evidence lies in observed species-specific mortality patterns. *Comfort* (1964), in his classical book *Ageing: the Biology of Senescence,* has thoroughly reviewed the evidence pertaining to this and has shown that differences of five orders of magnitude may be observed with respect to age and death (table I). Strain differences have also been observed within various species including *Drosophila* (*Pearl,* 1940), the mouse (*Grüneberg,* 1943; *Gowen,* 1962), the dog (*Comfort,* 1960, 1964), the horse (*Comfort,* 1962) and so on. Such evidence must, however, be analyzed and criticized from a strictly genetical point of view.

1. The Hereditary Basis of Ageing in Man

For obvious reasons, the basis of ageing and death in man has been thoroughly studied. Among the earliest researchers were *Beeton and Pearson* (1899, 1901) and the genealogist *Bell* (1918) who studied collections of genealogies. *Bell* made an analysis of the longevity of the descendants of William Hyde of Norwich, Conn., who died in 1681. When offspring or parents were classified into groups according to age at death, an almost direct relationship between the life-span of offspring and parents was indicated. More precisely, he showed that the average life-span of offspring whose parents had both died before the age of 60 was almost 20 years less than the average life-span of offspring whose parents lived more than 80 years (table II).

Table I. Maximum recorded longevities of different species of the animal kingdom

	Common name	Life-span	References
Vertebrate species			
Testudo sumeiri	Marion's tortoise	152 years	*Flower* (1937)
Testudo graeca	Greek tortoise	105 years	*Flower* (1937)
Elephas indicus	elephant	77 years	*Mohr* (1951)
Bubo bubo	eagle owl	68 years	*Flower* (1938)
Felis catus	domestic cat	31 years	*Mellen* (1940)
Colomba livia domestica	domestic pigeon	30 years	*Flower* (1938)
Mus musculus	laboratory mouse	3 years 5 months	*Kobozieff* (1931)
Invertebrate species			
Cervus pedunculatus (Coelenterata)		85–90 years	*Stephenson* (1935)
Homarus (Crustacea)		50 years	*Herrick* (1911)
Blaps gigas (Coleoptera)		imago: >10 years	*Labitte* (1916)
Porcellio scaber (Crustacea)		$3\frac{3}{4}$ years	*Collinge* (1944)
Maniola jurtina (Lepidoptera)		imago: 44 days	*Frohawk* (1935)
Epiphanes brachionus (Rotifers)		8 days	*Ferris* (1932)
Ephemera sp. (Ephemeroptera)		imago: from less than 2 h to 3 days	*Edmunds* (1965)

Table II. Mean longevity of man as a function of the age at death of the mother and the father. Age is indicated in years. Numbers in parentheses refer to sample size

Longevity of the father, years	Longevity of the mother, years		
	<60	60–80	>80
<60	32.8 (128)	33.4 (120)	36.3 (74)
60–80	35.8 (251)	38.0 (328)	45.0 (172)
>80	42.3 (131)	45.5 (206)	52.7 (184)

From *Bell* (1918).

Kallmann and his associates (*Kallmann et al.,* 1956; *Kallmann,* 1957) also showed that there was a consistent though small correlation of both maternal and paternal longevity with the longevity of both sons and daughters (table III). The effect of longevity in the two parents upon the longevity of the offspring is approximately additive although it is larger for sons than for daughters. That study was based upon the death records of twins and their siblings and was stimulated by the publication, in 1951, of a study on the inheritance of

Table III. Influence of the age at death of the parents on the mean longevity (in years) of twins and their siblings. Neither the estimates of the variation around the mean of the samples nor the size of the samples have been published

	Age at death of mother			Age at death of father			Age at death of parents		
	<55	55–70	>70	<55	55–70	>70	<55	55–70	>70
Sons	55.8	58.8	59.6	56.3	57.2	60.2	51.8	61.2	61.4
Daughters	64.8	64.0	66.4	63.0	64.3	65.3	62.1	61.7	66.8
Total	58.5	59.8	62.1	58.5	60.0	61.5	55.9	59.4	62.9

After *Kallmann* (1957).

longevity in mankind by *Jalavisto*. This author analyzed a set of family records of the Finnish and Swedish middle-class from the 16th to the 19th century. He did not consider births after 1829 in order to include only completed lines. A total number of 12,768 individuals were studied. When the offspring longevity is plotted as a function of the parental life-span, a linear regression is observed for the mother–offspring relationship (fig. 1), but a father–offspring relationship appears only in the case of sons and not of daughters.

Between 1945 and 1954, *Kallmann* collected an important sample of over 1,700 aged twin pairs residing in the state of New York. From his last known report, based on the life records of 78 monozygotic pairs and 102 dizygotic pairs, it appears that the mean intrapair differences vary, highly significantly, from 36.0 months for monozygotic twins to 74.6 for dizygotic twins of the same sex, whilst the intrapair difference for dizygotic twins of opposite sex reaches 106.0 months (table IV). It is a remarkable fact, according to the author, that monozygotic twins are more than twice as similar in causes of death as dizygotic twins of the same or opposite sex (*Kallmann and Sander*, 1948; *Kallmann*, 1957).

It is noteworthy that the relationship between parental and offspring longevity remains evident whatever the origin of the data. *Kallmann*'s team studied the longevity of aged twins born at the end of the 19th century, while

Fig. 1. A Relation between the life-span of daughters and sons and the life-span of the mother when the life-span of the father is held constant. *B* Relation between the life-span of daughters and sons and the life-span of the father when the life-span of the mother is held constant. Redrawn from *Jalavisto* (1951).

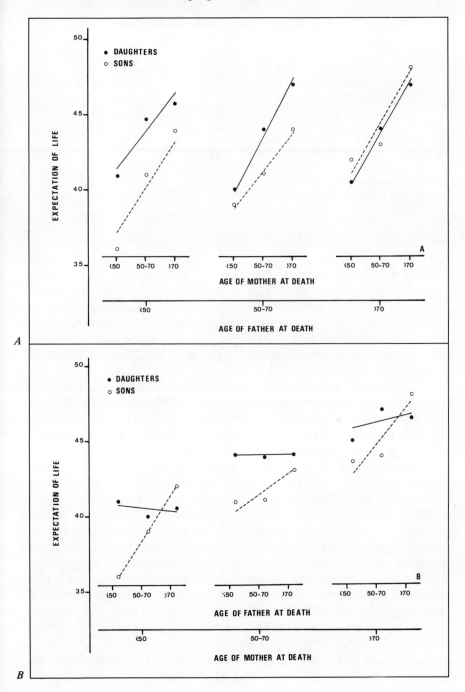

Table IV. Intra-pair differences in longevity (expressed in months) of human twins

Monozygotic	Male	40.7
	Female	31.6
	Total	36.0
Dizygotic	Male	69.5
	Female	79.1
	Total	74.6
Dizygotic	Male + female	106.0

After *Kallmann* (1957).

both *Jalavisto* and *Bell* analyzed a mixture of data from the early 16th to the early 19th century. The difference in expectation of life (due to decreased infantile mortality, better cures for illnesses of bacterial origin, eradication of epidemics and so on) for people born at such different times may probably be averaged at around 10–20 years; the mean longevity of offspring produced by parents who both died at more than 70 years of age is 45.7 years in *Jalavisto*'s study (calculated from fig. 1) and 52.7 years for offspring of parents who both died after 80 years in *Bell*'s study (table II), whilst it is 62.9 years in *Kallmann*'s analysis (table III).

Cohen (1964) wrote a highly critical review of all published evidence pertaining to the genetic basis of longevity in man. He classified the literature into two classes: (1) genealogical records – large individual kinships and collection of genealogies, and (2) samples from special subgroups of the population – working men's families, families of elderly persons, families of twins and an important subgroup comprising the families of insurees. According to *Cohen* most, if not all, of these studies suffer from one or both of the following defects: the statistical analysis is weak and the representativity of the chosen sample is questionable. Moreover, most of the investigations reviewed involve death which occurred in the pre-antibiotic and even the pre-public health era. However, taken together, we believe that the evidence resulting from that important review appears convincing. It may be summarized in a few words: people having long-lived parents have a greater life expectancy than people with short-lived parents. The conclusion of *Cohen* may therefore appear somewhat pessimistic, when he claims that: '...very little is known at present about the genetic aspects of longevity and mortality [in man]'. *Cohen* criticizes the technique but does not criticize the principle of the family analysis as a basis for ascertaining the genetic basis of ageing and death. Indeed, commenting on some preliminary results provided by an analysis of longevity in man started at the

John Hopkins University, he suggests that family patterns due to genetic factors, and probably with sex differences, emerge from the data so far collected. Such criticism, however, needs to be made.

2. Species and Strain Differences. Heritability

That there are species and strain differences in mean longevity is a point which should not be disputed. That among species and strains alike there are differences which, on the basis of comparisons between relatives, may be ascribed to *factors* common to those relatives is another point which is clearly established. Now these two types of evidence do not demonstrate either that the differences between species or strains nor that all or even part of the individual variations among species or strains are genetic in origin.

The argument on which the first assumption is based, namely that the differences in longevity between various species are genetic in origin, is quite simple, but wrong. It says that intrinsic mechanisms peculiar, for instance to *Drosophila, Mus* or *Homo* are responsible for the fact that a fruit-fly lives for some weeks, a mouse for some months and human beings for some years. Now, the argument proceeds, if the genetic constitution of *Drosophila*, mouse or human zygotes determines whether those zygotes will become *Drosophila*, mouse or man, and if each species has a characteristic life-span, it follows that the life-span is genetically determined.

The argument underlying the second assumption, namely that individual variations among species or strains are genetic in origin – and which, in turn, underlies the first assumption – relies on the results of calculations of correlations between the longevities of relatives, i.e. on the estimation of the heritability of the trait of longevity.

Heritability estimates the degree of resemblance between relatives, i.e. between parents and offspring, between brothers and sisters, between twins, and so on. It represents the proportion of the total phenotypic variation of a population which is ascribable to genetic variation. Thus, the heritability of a particular trait will be low when the environmental component of variance is high, and vice versa, of course. The genetic variation of a population or a strain is directly related to its genetic structure, as defined by a system of gene and genotype frequencies. It follows from it that the heritability of a trait is a property of a population at a precise moment of its history. When, for a given trait, a population is submitted to selection, which results in the modification of the genetic structure of the population, all the genetic variation of that population in respect to that trait will be exhausted after a certain time. At that time, the heritability of that particular trait becomes evidently equal to zero. However, this obviously does not mean that the trait is no more influenced by heredity; it means simply that none of the remaining variation in the population has a genetic origin. As stated by *Wallace* (1975) – though in relation to an entirely different topic — 'A difference in the average phenotypes of two populations need not have a genetic basis even though similar phenotypic variation *within* either or both populations is largely genetic in origin. Conversely, a difference in average phenotypes of two populations may have a genetic basis even though the heritability within each is zero!' It is therefore clear that heritability tells us nothing about the determinism of *inter*-strain differences.

What does heritability tell us about the determination of *intra*-group differences? As we have seen, the correlation coefficients between life-span of relatives are rather low. Besides, it is not impossible that even these low estimates are biased upwards simply because genotype and environment frequently fluctuate together rather than independently. This is particularly true for estimates based on twin data. But, on the other hand, it is not impossible that those estimates are biased downwards because the correlations between age and death of relatives generally do not take into account, or rather do not separate clearly, the senescent from the non-senescent deaths, due for instance to infectious diseases, car accidents or suicides. Impressive because of their recurrence, claims concerning the heredity of longevity based on heritability studies should certainly not be rejected; they should, however, be considered with caution.

The inadequacy of the analysis of family patterns as a definite proof of the genetic determinism of a given trait may be best illustrated by the recent history of kuru. Kuru is a mortal neurological disease which causes many deaths in the Fore, a tribe of the western part of New Guinea. For many years, on the basis of the study of family genealogies, the disease was ascribed to a dominant gene. It is now known from the Nobel Prize winning work of *Gajdusek* (*Gajdusek and Zigas,* 1957) that the disease is due to a very slowly reproducing viroid particle whose transmission from parent to offspring is due to a curious custom proper to the Fore tribe. More precisely, for more or less religious reasons, the members of that tribe regularly eat the brain, and eventually other parts, of a deceased parent. In this way, the agent responsible for the kuru disease is very simply transmitted by cannibalism.

3. Genetic Evidence
a. Major Genes
Now, are there any other genetic tests which may render the indirect evidence discussed above more obvious? We do not believe that the study of the influence of mutant major genes and of the combinations of such genes on the life-span of their carriers is likely to yield important results. It is highly probable that most, if not all, mutations of major genes have some effect on life-span, but it is doubtful whether the modifications in average life-span produced by such genes mimic in any respect the effects of normal ageing.

A constantly quoted analysis was made by *Gonzalez* (1923), a student of *Pearl.* He measured, in constant environmental conditions, the average life-span

Table V. Mean longevity of females and males of a wild strain and of homozygotic mutants and combinations of mutants of the chromosome II of *D. melanogaster* (in days)

Strain	Female	Male
Black	40.3 ± 0.5	41.1 ± 0.5
Purple	21.8 ± 0.2	27.4 ± 0.3
Vestigial	21.0 ± 0.4	15.0 ± 0.3
Arc	28.2 ± 0.4	25.2 ± 0.3
Speck	38.9 ± 0.6	46.6 ± 0.6
Black-purple	24.1 ± 0.3	30.4 ± 0.3
Black-vestigial	24.2 ± 0.4	16.4 ± 0.2
Black-arc	23.2 ± 0.4	20.1 ± 0.4
Black-speck	30.0 ± 0.3	32.4 ± 0.3
Purple-vestigial	19.0 ± 0.3	11.7 ± 0.1
Purple-arc	32.0 ± 0.4	36.0 ± 0.5
Purple-speck	23.0 ± 0.2	23.7 ± 0.2
Arc-speck	34.7 ± 0.7	38.4 ± 0.6
Quintuple mutant	12.1 ± 0.2	9.4 ± 0.2
Wild strain	40.6 ± 0.4	38.1 ± 0.4

Modified from *Gonzalez* (1923).

of the carriers of five mutations located on the chromosome II of *Drosophila melanogaster,* of eight double, six triple, three quadruple and the quintuple combination of those genes (table V). Large differences were observed, but the duration of life of various gene combinations is only rarely the average of the single mutations entering it. Deaths produced by major gene mutations, i.e. by modifications in the one or the other biosynthetic pathway are genetic accidents. His study may be of interest in showing that genetic accidents pertaining to life-span may exist, but we doubt that this will be of a great help in solving the problem of the natural variation in ageing. (We shall discuss later the problems raised by the study of single gene mutations in man which reduce life-span to a considerable extent, as for instance progeria or Werner's syndrome; p. 30). The variation in ageing present in natural populations and which is directly relevant to the problem of the determinism of ageing is variation of degree, not variation of kind.

b. Inbreeding and Crossbreeding
Better evidence as to the hereditary basis of ageing is, however, provided by experiments involving genetic manipulations, i.e. inbreeding and crossbreeding

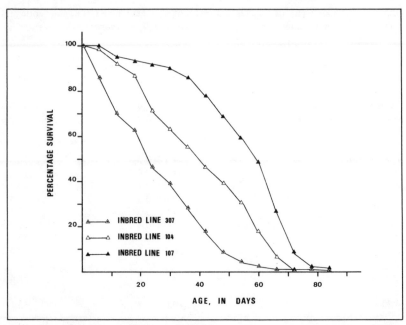

Fig. 2. D. melanogaster. Life-tables for two inbred lines – 104 and 107 – and an inbred line carrying the sepia mutation. The mean life-spans are 53.7 ± 1.1, 39.6 ± 0.7 and 25.2 ± 1.0 days for line 107, 104 and 307, respectively. Drawn from tables 5 and 6 in *Pearl and Parker* (1922a).

experiments. It should also be provided by selection experiments. Finally, differences in life-span related to sex should also be considered.

Inbreeding, i.e. reproduction through mates more or less closely related has two important genetic effects. When it is imposed on a normally outbreeding population, that population is broken up into smaller groups, into lines. These lines diverge genetically from each other and in each of them the progress of inbreeding is accompanied by an increase in genetic fixation, i.e. in the degree of homozygosity. Inbreeding leads generally, but not necessarily, to a loss of fitness, referred to as inbreeding depression. The absence, presence and amount of depression is linked to the type – deleterious or not – and number of genes fixed in the line (fig. 2; table VIII).

When inbred lines are crossed together, the hybrid progeny generally display heterosis, i.e. superiority with respect to one or more characters by comparison with the corresponding inbred lines or even with the natural population(s) from which the inbred lines were issued. Heterosis could be due to heterozygosity *per se,* also called overdominance, i.e. the fact that at any given locus the hetero-zygous combination of two genes is superior in fitness to either of the possible

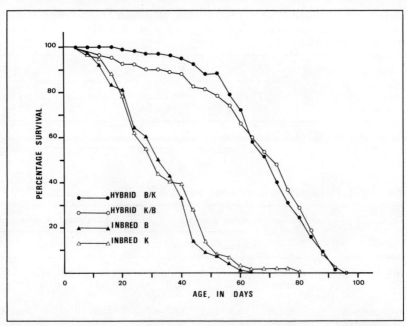

Fig. 3. In *D. subobscura* the mean life-span of hybrids, B/K and K/B, is approximately twice that of inbreds, B and K. Redrawn with permission from *Clarke and Maynard Smith* (1955).

homozygotes. The hybrid having relatively favourable dominant alleles at more different loci than is the case for either inbred, heterosis could also be due to ordinary dominance of genes which are relatively favourable and corresponding recessivity of genes unfavourable for fitness. The precise causes of heterosis are still disputed although nobody disputes the genetic nature of that determinism.

Clarke and Maynard Smith (1955) studied the longevity, at 19 °C, of two lines of *D. subobscura* previously inbred for 14 generations, and of the hybrids obtained from reciprocal crosses made between those two lines. The expectation of life at emergence for the two hybrid strains is approximately twice that of inbred flies (fig. 3, table VI). In mice, a species which is much less sensible to inbreeding depression than *Drosophila*, confirmation of these results was provided by *Mühlbock* (1959) who compared the mean longevity of two inbred strains of mice — DBA$_f$, mean = 20.3 months; O$_{20}$, mean = 22.4 months — with the longevity of the hybrid strain O$_{20}$ × DBA$_f$, mean = 24.1 months (the means have been calculated from fig. 4).

Similar results have been obtained in *D. melanogaster* by *Hyde* (1913) and *Pearl and Parker* (1922a, b), in a study of nine inbred lines and four outbred

Table VI. D. subobscura. Mean longevity (in days) of males and females of two inbred lines (B and K) and of the two reciprocal hybrids (B × K and K × B) issued from the crosses between the inbred lines

Strain	B	K	B × K	K × B
Male	27.7 ± 1.9	39.2 ± 2.1	63.4 ± 2.4	67.3 ± 2.9
Female	35.1 ± 1.8	25.0 ± 1.5	70.6 ± 2.4	62.0 ± 3.2

After *Clarke and Maynard Smith* (1955).

Table VII. The longevities of inbred and outbred *D. subobscura*, in days, at 20 °C

		Mean longevity		Coefficient of variation	
		female	male	female	male
Nine inbred lines	Range	17.2–53.8	17.1–69.2	0.35–0.69	0.35–0.66
	Mean	36.4	40.0	0.51	0.55
Four outbred populations	Range	55.9–64.1	44.7–67.4	0.29–0.35	0.23–0.50
	Mean	60.0	56.8	0.32	0.33

From *Maynard Smith* (1959).

strains – hybrids and offspring flies caught in the wild – in *D. subobscura* (table VII) (*Maynard Smith*, 1959), and in mice by *Gates* (1926). *Comfort* (1964) reported hybrids from a cross between goldfinches and canaries that had a greater longevity than their parents.

c. Selection

Artificial selection is a purposeful process of differential and non-random reproduction of different phenotypes. Its goal is to change permanently the specific phenotypic characters of a population. Its success depends on the correspondence between phenotype and genotype. When that correspondence is high, the response to selection will be equally high. When it is low or non-existent, the response will be equally small or non-existent. We did note that the phenotypic variability of a population need not have a genetic basis.

The effectiveness of selection for a given trait in producing a response in a previously unselected population thus depends on the amount of genetic variability in the population. We know of no experimental results showing a successful selection for prolonged life-span. For years, however, most reviewers

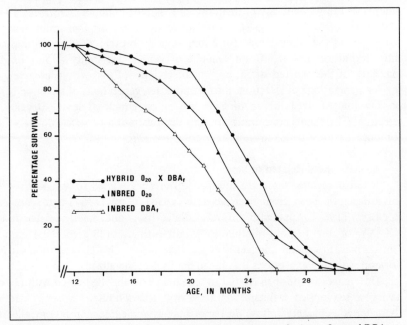

Fig. 4. Survival curves of the females of two inbred strains of mice – O_{20} and DBA$_f$ – and their F$_1$ hybrids – O_{20} × DBA$_f$. Redrawn with permission from *Mühlbock* (1959).

credited *Strong* (1936) with having demonstrated, by selection, the existence of a certain amount of genetic variability affecting life-span among an experimental mouse colony. The original text of 1936 says the following: *'Up to 2 years ago,* spontaneous tumours in mice belonging to the *inbred* CBA strain were extremely rare. The strain had been produced primarily by a *brother-to-sister mating since 1920.* On account of this rarity of spontaneous tumours, a *selection experiment toward longevity* was set up. This procedure was followed since it was obvious that for a strain of mice to be highly resistant to spontaneous tumours, the mice ought to live well beyond the age variability of the common types of spontaneous tumours in that species of animals. Since carcinoma of the female mammary gland and carcinoma of the male lung are the commonest types of tumours found in mice and since these manifest themselves on an average of 10–12 and 14–16 months, respectively, it became highly desirable to have resistant mice live considerably beyond this age period. In the present selection experiment, only *the descendants of that mouse in each generation which lived longest* were continued. *By 1930,* an *inbred* strain had been obtained, the individuals of which, in direct descent *for 10 generations,* averaged more than 24 months of life without any of them showing signs of tumours ...' (*Strong,* 1936) (italics ours). No data are given on the longevity of the original strain – which was apparently a strain inbred for a long time by brother X sister matings and thus devoid of any significant amount of genetic variability – nor on the longevity of the selected strain, nor on the changes of longevity accompanying the ten generations of selection. Furthermore, ten generations of selection based on the longest lived mouse of each generation entails at least 20 years of selection! The claims concerning *Strong*'s demonstration of successful selection for longevity must be taken *cum (enormo) grano salis.*

d. Differences Related to Sex

In most species, there are life-span differences related to sex. Reviews on this topic have been given by *Rockstein* (1958), *Clark* (1964) and *Clark and Rockstein* (1964). Apparently, however, longevity is not directly related to the XX–XY or the haploid–diploid state, although according to some authors females have in general a longer life-span than males. This last assertion suffers, however, so many exceptions that it can hardly be generalized.

Differences in life-span related to sex could probably be related with factors having a sex-limited influence on longevity. A sex-limited or sex-controlled character is a character whose degree of phenotypic expression is controlled by the sexual condition of the individual. The sex controls or modifies the expression of the character, but not the chromosomal transmission of the hereditary determinant, with the exception, of course, of the heterosomes. That longevity is sex-controlled to some extent may be shown by the comparison of female and male longevities in various strains. *Maynard Smith* (1959), in *D. subobscura,* studied the longevity of females and males of nine inbred lines, of two F_1 hybrid strains between inbred lines and of the offspring of two groups of females caught in the wild (table VIII). In eight of the 13 populations, there is a significant difference between the longevities of the two sexes, but in four cases it is the males and in four cases the females which live longer. This is a good indication of the presence of genes which affect longevity of the two sexes differently. An even better demonstration emerges from another study of *Maynard Smith* (1959), who calculated the correlations between the longevities of relatives in a population derived from females caught in the wild in Galilee (table IX). The coefficients of correlation are rather low. This is not new and means that many differences between members of the population are due to uncontrolled, unknown or intangible variations of the environment in the largest sense of the word. The important point for the present discussion is that all the correlations between relatives of like sex are positive and significant, whereas only one of the four correlations between relatives of unlike sex is significantly different from zero. These experimental findings should of course be compared with similar results found by *Jalavisto, Kallmann* and others in humans.

Table VIII. Longevity of males and females of various inbred, hybrid and wild strains of *D. subobscura,* in days, at 20 °C; ratio between female and male longevity. Of the nine inbred lines the K line was derived from flies caught at Küssnacht in Switzerland, the B, NFS and O lines from individual females caught in southern England and the D, E, F, G and M lines from flies caught at Edinburgh in Scotland

	Longevity		Ratio	p
	female	male		
Inbred lines				
K	17.2	31.2	0.55	**
M	35.3	51.8	0.68	*
F	53.8	69.2	0.77	*
O	48.7	52.5	0.93	
NFS	40.7	42.4	0.98	
D	50.2	47.5	1.06	
B	33.3	25.8	1.29	*
G	30.0	22.6	1.33	*
E	36.2	17.1	2.12	**
F₁ hybrids				
K × NFS	55.9	67.4	0.83	**
B × K	61.5	61.6	1.00	
Offspring of wild flies				
Kent	58.6	53.4	1.10	
Galilee	64.1	44.7	1.43	**

From *Maynard Smith* (1959).
* Significant at 0.10 level.
** Significant at 0.001 level.

Table IX. Correlations between the longevities of relatives among the descendants of *D. subobscura* females caught in the wild in Galilee

Like sex			Unlike sex		
Brother-brother	F_1	0.13			
Brother-brother	F_2	0.19			
			Brother-sister	F_1	0.04
			Brother-sister	F_2	0.04
Sister-sister	F_1	0.12			
Sister-sister	F_2	0.20			
Father-son		0.29	Father-daughter		0.19
Mother-daughter		0.15	Mother-son		−0.04

From *Maynard Smith* (1959).

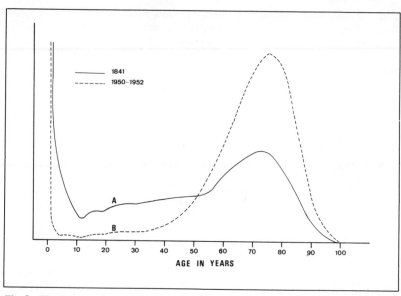

Fig. 5. The comparison of the curves of deaths for english males, based on the life-tables of 1841 (A) and 1950–52 (B), shows that in the past hundred years or so the peak in the age distribution in the general male population of England has slightly moved to a more advanced age – from 72 to 76 years – and, importantly, that the percentage of deaths occurring at an early age and which on the basis of simple assumptions might be regarded as non-senescent deaths, has been drastically reduced – from about 60 to about 30%. Redrawn from figures 1 and 3 in *Benjamin* (1959).

4. Life-Span. A Hereditary Trait

This rapid survey of the evidence in favour of the hereditary basis of ageing shows that there are some good reasons for accepting that life-span is, to a certain extent, an hereditary trait. It is, however, almost impossible to be more precise. Indeed, in a given species, deaths which occur at various ages may be considered to be due to causes intrinsic or extrinsic to the species under consideration. Intrinsic causes are linked to the normal differentiation and development of the well-balanced individual of that species; they are pro-grammed. Genetic – and thus programmed – accidents leading to an early death, due to gross chromosomal or genic mutations, constitute a special case; because of our definition of intrinsic causes, we are tempted to classify them among extrinsic factors.

Other causes extrinsic to the species are, for instance, infectious diseases, accidents – car crashes for human beings, predation for dogs and cats – and so on. In other words, there are senescent and non-senescent deaths, a distinction which was clearly stated by *Clarke* (1950) (*Benjamin, 1959*).

In human populations, it is highly probable that modern medical care and various social approaches to human welfare will to a large extent diminish or even eradicate the proportion of non-senescent deaths (fig. 5). A better under-standing of the biology of laboratory animals and improvement in the breeding methods might also be expected to increase the relative percentage of senescent deaths in laboratory strains submitted to experimentation. It follows that studies using pure genetic tests could in the future yield clearer and more precise results than the rare ones obtained up to now.

A last point should be stressed. The demonstration that ageing and death in a large series of different species are genetically determined, should, by no means, signify that death and ageing are in those species controlled by identical or even similar mechanisms. The ways in which organisms differentiate, grow and develop are so numerous and so different that there is every reason to suspect that ageing could follow very different paths leading to the ultimate step in differentiation, i.e. death.

Anyhow, if one accepts an hereditary basis of ageing and death − and I do not see how that point could be disputed − it appears as a strange paradox that for the last 20 years the causes of ageing have not been searched for at the level of a positive or negative control through the switching in or out, at appropriate times, of a given set of information, but have been claimed to be due to a series of purely stochastic events.

B. The Mutation Theory of Ageing

Among others (*Failla*, 1958; *Szilard*, 1959), *Curtis and Gebhard* proposed in 1958 that ageing and death were due to the accumulation of a certain number of somatic mutations. Says *Curtis* (1966): 'According to this theory, the somatic cells of the body develop spontaneous mutations in the same way as do the germ cells. Once a mutation has been formed, subsequent cell divisions will perpetuate it. As more and more cells develop mutations, the time comes when an appre- ciable fraction of the cells is mutated. Practically all mutations are deleterious, so the cells carrying mutations are less well able to perform their functions. The organs become inefficient and senescent.' The major argument in favour of the theory apparently resided in the fact that, at least in mammals, radiation − which provokes various chromosomal damage − induces, or at least accelerates, the development of degenerative diseases (*Henshaw et al.*, 1947; *Stevenson and Curtis*, 1961; *Curtis*, 1963; *Curtis and Crowley*, 1963). A minor objection to this view was that if the number of mutations in the somatic cells is the same as it is in the germ cells, that number seemed inadequate to account for senescence. An answer to that objection was given by assuming that the mutation rate in somatic cells could be 10−12 times larger that in germ cells (*Failla*, 1958).

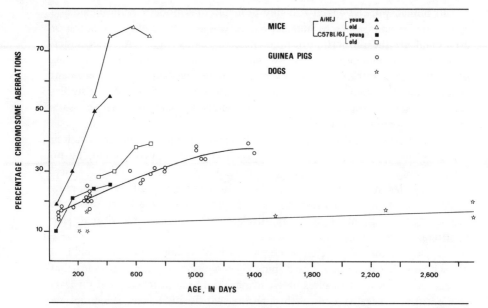

Fig. 6. Percentage of chromosomal aberrations measured in cells of regenerating livers as a function of age for three different species: mice, guinea pigs and dogs. Two strains of mice have been used in the experiments, strain A/HEJ which has a life expectancy of 395 days and strain C57BL/6J which has a life expectancy of 600 days. The mean life-span of guinea pigs is of about 6 years, and that of the beagle dogs used in the experiments is of 12 years. Redrawn with permission from *Crowley and Curtis* (1963), *Curtis et al.* (1966) and *Curtis and Miller* (1971).

1. Mutations and Ageing. In vivo *Observations*

Evidence concerning the mutation theory of ageing was claimed to have been obtained from the observation of the number of chromosome aberrations in cells from regenerating livers of various mammal species. The justification for relating this quantity to the numbers of mutations comes, according to the authors, from the work of *Caldecott* (1961) with plants. In plants, somatic cells eventually differentiate to form germinal cells whose mutations may be scored. *Caldecott* found, under a wide variety of circumstances, that the number of mutations is proportional to the chromosome aberrations of these somatic cells. For *Curtis and Miller* (1971), the inverse relation between spontaneous chromosome aberration rate and normal life expectancy of three different species, namely mice, guinea pigs and dogs (fig. 6), constitutes therefore a good proof in favour of the mutation theory. The consideration of that particular set of data leads, however, to ask a certain number of questions which, as far as we know, have not been answered. Let us recall that the mutation theory assumed that ageing is caused by the gradual accumulation of spontaneous mutations in the somatic cells of the body. This renders the organs inefficient, senescent and eventually leads the organism to death.

A first question then sounds: Why does a mouse accumulate in a given time 5—8 times more aberrations than a dog (fig. 6)? Should this mean that the average mutation rate per gene of the mouse genome is so much higher than the average mutation rate of the dog? Almost all mammalian diploid cells having similar DNA content (*Sober,* 1970), there is no obvious reason to make such an assumption. *Szilard* (1959), however, in a highly theoretical approach to the mutation theory, assumed such a postulate. Says *Szilard:* 'We further assume that the rate at which chromosomes of a somatic cell suffer such "hits" is a characteristic of the species ...' This may appear contradictory to a preceding sentence of the same paper: 'We assume that "aging hits" are random events and that the probability that a chromosome of a somatic cell suffers such a "hit" per unit of time remains constant throughout life.'

A second and more important question bears to the fact that, according to the data presented in figure 6, a low number of chromosomal aberrations is sufficient to kill a dog whilst a great number of them is necessary to kill a mouse! In this connection, it is difficult to understand why dogs are dying at a relatively advanced age whilst the recorded amount of chromosomal aberrations remains almost constant during their entire life-span. Nothing in the mutation theory, as it stands, may explain such oddities. We guess that a much better argument in favour of the importance of mutations in the ageing phenomenon would be provided by the demonstration that, for various species, ageing and death occur when approximately the same amount of chromosomal aberrations has been attained. Such a demonstration has, of course, never been given.

2. Mutations and Ageing. In vitro *Observations*

Recent evidence provided by *Hart and Setlow* (1974) could eventually explain why a mouse does accumulate such a high percentage of chromosomal aberrations or, at least, why that percentage is so much higher in mice than in dogs. This, however, does absolutely not explain why death occurs for a mouse when 80% of its cells contain chromosomal aberrations whilst 10% aberrant cells are enough to kill a dog. *Hart and Setlow* measured for seven species the ability of fibroblasts in culture to perform, after UV irradiation, unscheduled DNA synthesis, i.e. the synthesis of DNA during the non-S period of the cell — a measure of excision repair. They observe a good correlation between both the rate and the extent of unscheduled DNA synthesis and the logarithm of the life-span of the species — shrew, mouse, rat, hamster, cow, elephant, mare. Now, as noted by the authors, it is possible, but not certain that unscheduled DNA synthesis mimics somehow or other what may happen in a cell as a function of the normal wear and tear of cellular DNA, but it is by no means certain that there is any relation between excision repair and life-span. For instance, patients suffering from xeroderma pigmentosum are defective in excision repair (*Setlow et al.*, 1969; *Bootsma et al.*, 1970). Such individuals develop sunlight-induced skin cancers from which they would die if untreated; but such individuals do not age in any other way, nor do they have a life-span shorter than that of a mouse. Furthermore, cultures of fibroblasts from such patients do not go through a fewer number of passages (p. 26) than normal ones. Finally, fibroblasts from patients suffering from progeria, and who age and die prematurely, do not go through as many passages as do normal cells (*Martin et al.*, 1970), but they show normal level of excision repair (*Cleaver*, 1970; *Regan and Setlow*, 1974). That last point is, however, equivocal since other authors (*Epstein et al.*, 1973, 1974) obtained data indicating that fibroblasts from individuals with progeroid symptoms were defective in their ability to repair single-strand breaks in their DNA.

Recently, using the double-label autoradiography technique, *Hart and Setlow* (1976) measured both scheduled DNA synthesis – a measure of the amount of cells going through an S-period – and unscheduled DNA synthesis after UV irradiation – a measure of excision repair – in W1-38 cells from passage 18 to passage 60. Late passage cells showed less repair than early passage cells and many of them showed none. But the authors showed that there was a good correlation between cells that do scheduled synthesis and cells that do unscheduled synthesis. In other words, a cell that does not do scheduled synthesis is unlikely to do unscheduled synthesis. Furthermore, the decrease of unscheduled synthesis with passage number is slower than of scheduled synthesis. The authors, therefore, interpret their results as indicating that failure of repair is *not* a causal event in the failure of late passage cells to divide.

3. Objections to the Theory. Genetic Redundancy

We think that the major objection to the mutation theory of ageing came from some elegant experimental evidence provided by *Clark and Rubin* (1961) and *Clark et al.* (1963). The wasp *Habrobracon serinopae* produces both haploid and diploid males. When haploid and diploid males are treated by X-rays, the decrease of life-span observed is related to chromosomal damage brought about by irradiation; the decrease observed in haploids is larger than that observed in diploids. Now the somatic mutation theory implies that in non-irradiated animals haploid males should have a shorter life-span than diploids, simply because the haploids lack the genetic redundancy of the diploids. In fact, such haploid and diploid males have identical life-span. In view of those data, *Curtis* (1966) attempted to save the somatic mutation theory by assuming that senescence in mammals and in 'lower forms of animal life such as insects' is essentially a different phenomenon, 'somatic mutations play(ing) little, if any, role in aging in adult insects'.

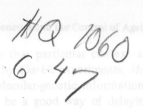

notwithstanding the type of evidence pro-
vided by such mutants. *Medvedev* (1972, 1975) suggested that repetition
of molecular-genetic information, i.e. the redundancy of some types of genes,
could be a good way of delaying ageing and increasing longevity. He further
suggested that such repetition could possibly be a factor acting during the
evolutionary changes of life-span. Says *Medvedev:* '... if accumulation of molecular alterations has any importance for slow ageing of highly differentiated cells,
the limiting factors of life-span have to be located in parts of the cellular
metabolizing system which are coded by unique genes or unique templates. [...]
The life-span evolution of whose organisms [...] may depend on the total supply
of non-repeated information in the genome and in the specialized structures of
the body. Increasing proportion of non-repeated unique information means [...]
the shortening of life-span.'

First of all, it must be noted that the redundancy of important genes has
never been clearly demonstrated, except of course for rRNA, histones (*Kedes
and Birnstiel,* 1971) and tRNA (*Quincey and Wilson,* 1969) genes, whose special
role during development is well known. In the duck, *Bishop et al.* (1972)
estimated that there were about five globin genes per genome, but the experimental conditions leading to that estimate were criticized (Anonymous,
1972). Examining those data and criticisms, as well as their own data on the
globin genes in the mouse genome, *Harrison et al.* (1972) consider that the most
likely model which emerges is that each globin mRNA is transcribed from a
single locus. *Cutler* (1973/74) did not demonstrate, but estimated – and that
estimation is based on a series of highly speculative assumptions – that genes
involved in transcription of mRNA in the brain tissue of mice, cows and humans
increased by an average redundancy value of 1.3, 1.5 and 2.1, respectively!

More fundamentally, however, the thesis of redundancy of information
content in the genome as a protective mechanism determining ageing rate – a
thesis adopted by *Cutler* (1973/74) for the mammalian species only – suffers
from a certain number of internal contradictions. What does that thesis affirm?
It affirms that modifications in the information content of a cell result in
defective proteins which, somehow or other, have the effect of reducing life-
span. Furthermore, and following *Cutler,* the mutation – a random process! –
could be an important factor in the production of such defective proteins.

Two objections come to mind. Firstly, ageing and death are apparently not
random, as the simple consideration of the species-specific life-span may suggest.
If this is admitted, the following paradox emerges: a non-random process –
ageing and death – is explained in terms of a random-process-mutation! Says
Cutler: 'If there are only a few major ageing processes, then they would
necessarily have to act at a very fundamental level associated with the ageing
process and to be able to be related at a common level to the degeneration of
many diverse physiological functions and the causes of many similarly diverse

degenerative diseases. A process that appears sufficiently fundamental to satisfy these conditions and which is likely to be *controllable* (italics ours) by a relatively small number of genes is the production of defective proteins.' I wonder how such a fundamentally correct view may be reconciled with the idea of detrimental defective proteins produced by mutations.

Secondly, it may be asked, more essentially, to what an extent genetic redundancy, instead of being a protective device, is not, on the contrary, a severe load. Indeed, the more a gene is repeated, the more chances there are that one or the other of these repetitions is mutated. Corollarily, the more chances there are that these mutated genes produce proteins, which are more or less similar to the one produced by the non-mutated normal gene. A thesis may then easily be defended which says that an increase in the redundancy of essential genes will increase the probability to see essential metabolic pathways partially or totally inactivated or, at the worst, transformed by the products of the mutated genes. Redundancy would then result in a decreased life-span. *Cutler* does not totally ignore that objection since he writes: 'The redundancy of genes could theoretically decrease the frequency of defective protein production by insuring the presence of a minimum number of mutation-free genes. However, in order for this protective mechanism to operate; *a means must be available either to inactivate the mutated gene or to eliminate the defective protein it produces*' (italics ours). One may guess, however, that such a means could hardly proceed from a random process. In other words, if such a means did exist, it could be interpreted in favour of a mutation theory of senescence only with difficulty. Indeed, longevity would not then appear as the result of a series of stochastic events. Rather, it would appear as the outcome of an evolutionary directed genome restructuration or built-in enzymatic system of DNA damage repair or defective proteins degradation. *Goldberg* (1972), for instance, found evidence that *Escherichia coli* contains a mechanism for selective degradation of abnormal proteins. He too holds that such a mechanism could not have appeared and evolved except under the influence of a strong selective pressure due to the highly deleterious intracellular accumulation of inactive or partially active enzymes. That last point — and more precisely the presence or absence of partially active enzymes in ageing organisms — will, however, be further discussed (p. 37).

C. The Error-Catastrophe Theory of Ageing

The deficiencies of the mutation theory meant the necessity for further research. In 1963, *Orgel* proposed a theory which rapidly became known as the protein-error or error-catastrophe theory. Says *Orgel:* 'The basic idea is a simple one, namely that the ability of a cell to produce its complement of functional proteins depends not only on the correct genetic specification of the various polypeptide sequences, but also on the competence of the protein-synthetic apparatus. A cell inherits, in addition to its genetic DNA, the enzymes necessary for the transcription of that material into polypeptide sequences ... A cell may deteriorate through a progressive decrease in the adequacy of its transcription mechanism, just as it may through the accumulation of somatic mutations.' He further argues that for the majority of enzymes the presence of a few defective molecules would result merely in a slight lowering of the metabolic efficiency, but that this would not be so for that group of enzymes which is necessary for transcription or translation. Finally, he claims that he is *not* proposing that the accumulation of protein transcription errors is the mechanism of ageing. However, he suggests to test the theory by increasing errors in protein synthesis in microorganisms or in mice by treating them with appropriate amino acid analogues.

When applied, as it was suggested and done, to ageing and death of organisms, it should be noted that the error-catastrophe theory of ageing is nothing else than a modified version of the mutation theory. More essentially, it reflects the same basic attitude versus the determinism of ageing. Indeed, in both cases one or a series of random events cause the cells to perform syntheses of inaccurate and damageable proteins or to stop the syntheses of adequate proteins. The *deus ex machina* is random, the primary events are different, the end-results identical. In the mutation theory, the primary event is a badly coded DNA and in the error-catastrophe theory it lies in the malfunctioning of the protein-synthetic apparatus, at the level either of transcription or of translation.

A general remark may be made at this level. Theories which rest on random events, whose probabilities may, however, be estimated (the rate of mutation of a great number of genes is known, the probability of error frequency during the synthesis of mRNA has been estimated, and so on) appear to be unable to explain the enormous differences in life-span of the living organisms, not even the large differences which may exist between closely related species. Suppose that ageing and death are due to a bad functioning of the cell or of groups of cells and that there is a common process of deterioration – mutation! error-catastrophe! – of the harmonious functioning of the cells. Hence, at least for nearly related species, individuals should age and die at relatively identical rates. This is not so. The causes of ageing thus differentiate the organisms. It therefore appears reasonable to look at the causes of ageing at the level of the protective devices against ineluctable errors, which happen with known frequencies. The deterioration or blocking of such devices may allow the expression of the consequences of these errors. The protective devices of various organisms, at the evidence, function for very different periods of time; therefore, they could be either identical but differently programmed, or as diverse of the organisms. In other words, even if the mutations postulated by the mutation-theory, or the primary error in protein synthesis postulated by the error-catastrophe theory, do have deleterious effects on the functioning of cells and/or cell lines, this is absolutely not enough to explain species-specific longevities.

1. Pros

Confirmation of one of *Orgel*'s main predictions was given in 1967 by *Harrison and Holliday*. *Drosophila melanogaster* larvae were fed with various amino acid analogues or with streptomycin in order to increase artificially the frequency of mistakes in protein synthesis. Such a treatment does indeed decrease the life-span of adults. (These experiments have been repeated in slightly different environmental conditions and yielded contradictory results; p. 35). However, the experiment of *Harrison and Holliday* suffers the same basic defect as some experiments of *Curtis* designed to test the validity of the mutation theory of ageing. The theories say that ageing is due to mutations (to incompetence of the protein-synthetic apparatus), radiation increases mutations (amino acid analogues increase the frequency of errors in protein synthesis) and decreases life-span; thus, ageing and longevity are due to mutations (to a protein-error catastrophe). This kind of circular argument ignores the fact that radiation and amino acid analogues are not necessarily part of the normal life either of man, mouse or *Drosophila*.

Orgel's hypothesis, however, received further although apparently still inconclusive confirmation (*Holliday*, 1975) through a series of experimental evidence provided by *Holliday* and co-workers working essentially *in vitro* on a variety of cell cultures.

a. Note on the Relevance to the Ageing Problem of the Study of Cell Strain Cultures *in vitro*

In recent years, the study of cell strain cultures of various origin has taken a great importance in laboratories engaged in gerontological research. It is therefore useful to see to what an extent such studies are entirely relevant to the study of ageing. Most of these researches have been realized on fibroblasts or fibroblast-like cells. Fibroblasts are the principal and most characteristic cells of non-rigid connective tissues. They are large cells with an elongated form having processes extending out from the cell body. They produce the major component of the collagen fibril.

Until 15 or 20 years ago, it was generally thought that *in vitro* fibroblast cultures could proliferate indefinitely. This assumption was based on the studies of *Carrel* and some of his students just after the first world war (*Ebeling*, 1913; *Carrel and Ebeling*, 1921). *Swim and Parker* (1957) showed that this assumption was wrong when they demonstrated that 51 strains of human fibroblasts of various origins could only be cultivated for a limited period of time. Later on, *Hayflick and Moorhead* (1961) demonstrated essentially the same thing. More precisely, they have shown that normal embryonic diploid cell strains in culture

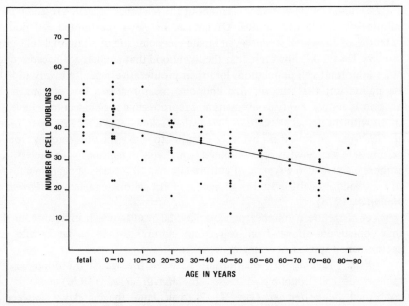

Fig. 7. Relation between age of donor at biopsy and number of cell doublings achieved by human skin fibroblasts. The equation of the regression calculated by the method of the least squares for the entire set of data – including fetal biopsies – is of the form y = 43.84 – 0.21x. The correlation coefficient equals r = – 0.55 (n = 95) which means that 31% of the variance is ascribable to a linear relationship. One must be aware that this regression means that a number of zero cell doublings will be attained by donors aged 211 years. It may equally be noted that *Schneider and Chase* (1976) calculated a regression taking only into account the data from the second to the ninth decade of life, arguing that human ageing may be defined as the period from puberty to death. This last regression is significant but only 11.7% of the variance is ascribable to the linear regression. Recalculated and redrawn with permission from *Martin et al.* (1970).

multiply actively during a period which is generally less than 1 year. Thereafter, these cells demonstrate an increased doubling time, gradual cessation of mitotic activity, accumulation of cellular debris and ultimately total degeneration of the culture.

More recently (*Martin et al.,* 1970), the culture of fibroblasts derived from biopsies of a hundred people ranging from fetal to 90 years of age, showed that there is a precise negative correlation between the age of the donor at biopsy and the number of cell doublings (fig. 7). Very precisely, the equation of the regression relating number of cell doublings to age is the following: Y = 43.84–0.21X, which means that there is a decrement of 0.21 population doublings per year of donor life. The significance of the regression is very high, and unquestionable.

Hayflick (1973) was very clear about the relevance to ageing research of the culture of diploid cell strains. Of course, he views the limited cell doubling potential of these cell strains as an innate characteristic of all normal cells grown *in vitro*. He thinks, however, that the likelihood that animals age because one or more important cell populations lose their proliferative capacity is very unlikely. He points out that the *in vitro* endpoint measured as a loss of capacity for division is simply a very convenient and reproducible system but may have little to do with the actual cause of *in vivo* ageing. Likewise, in a recent paper, *Linn et al.* (1976) admit that it is obviously essential to verify the observations from cell culture senescence with cells obtained from living organisms. Nevertheless, some authors claim that the system of cultured human fibroblasts appears increasingly to be a valid model for studies of ageing of the whole organism (*Goldstein and Moerman,* 1976).

Yet there are a number of experimental results which undoubtedly show that conclusions drawn from cell strain cultures should be taken with great caution when applied to ageing in organisms.

Firstly. The *negative* relationship between the age of the donor and the number of cell doublings disclosed by *Martin et al.* (1970) has not been confirmed. *Schneider and Chase* (1976) calculated the regression between donor's age and number of cell doublings for eight cultures originated from adults aged between 26 and 87 years (data from *Hayflick,* 1965). The regression is *positive* but insignificant. It must, however, be noted that a complementary statistical analysis made on *Hayflick*'s data reveals a highly significant difference in the onset of phase III (the begin of the degeneration period of the culture) in fetal cultures, 48.2 ± 2.2 cell doublings, and in adult cultures, 20.5 ± 1.7. The same study by *Schneider and Chase* reveals that the *in vitro* life-span of skin fibroblast cultures derived from normal donors (data from *Goldstein et al.,* 1969) is negatively correlated with donor's age, but that the regression is *non*-significant.

Secondly. The replicative life-span of human fibroblasts is a function of the tissue of origin. In the case of explants obtained from the same individuals, there is a far greater replicative life-span of cells derived from skin than from skeletal muscle, from skeletal muscle than from bone marrow spicules. Reasons for these differences are not known. They may reflect differences in the previous *in vivo* history of the cells, such as a precise pattern of differentiation or a previous replication history (*Martin et al.,* 1970).

Thirdly. The life-span of human embryonic cell strain cultures treated with cortisone – a hormone which, among others, controls the metabolism of mesenchymal tissue *in vivo* (*Castor and Baker,* 1950) – is increased. With respect to the controls cultivated in the classical medium (*Eagle,* 1955), the increase varies between 25 and 35% (*Macieira-Coelho,* 1966). These results have been extended by *Cristofalo and Kabakjian* (1975), who showed that the presence of

Table X. The relation between maximum life-span and number or range of cell doublings

Species	Maximum life-span years	Number or range of cell-doublings	References
Homo sapiens	105	35–55	*Martin et al.* (1970)
Equus caballus	46	82	*Stanley et al.* (1975)
Macaca speciosa	34	60	*Stanley et al.* (1975)
Felis catus	31	92	*Stanley et al.* (1975)
Gallus domesticus	30	15–35	*Hay and Strehler* (1967) *Ponten* (1970) *Macieira-Coelho and Lima* (1973)
Macropus gigantus	16	46*	*Stanley et al.* (1975)
Oryctolagus cuniculus	13	70*	*Stanley et al.* (1975)
Mus musculus	3.5	14–28	*Todaro and Green* (1963) *Rothfels et al.* (1963)
Sminthopsis crassicaudata	3	170	*Stanley et al.* (1975)

Maximum life-span: from *Comfort* (1964), *Collins* (1973) and Biology Data Book (1972). All cell strains originated from fetal or new-born tissues except the ones marked * which are derived from adult tissues.

hydrocortisone in the culture medium extended the life-span of the W1-38 cell strain by 20–30%. This may explain that some investigators still believe that the limited potential of division of normal cells in culture is an artefact and why they claim that with an appropriate environment normal cells would divide forever. That view is reinforced by some recent data of *Packer and Smith* (1974) and *Packer and Fuehr* (1977). The first study has shown that the addition of vitamin E to cultured human fibroblasts of the W1-38 strain (and the use of a special lot of fetal serum) increases the *in vitro* life-span of these cells from 50 to 120 population doublings. The second study relates to the growth and life-span of two human diploid cell strains, W1-38 and IMR-90. They indeed showed that growth is enhanced at oxygen concentration less than 20% and that an extension of about 25% of the life-span of both cell types is realized by long-term cultivation under 10% oxygen.

Fourthly. A relation between the final doubling numbers achieved by cultured diploid cells and the life-span of the animal species from which the cells were derived has been suggested (*Hayflick,* 1973). Such a relation does probably *not* exist (table X).

Finally, one should note that these reserves are most probably not shared by all gerontologists. There is a certain number of arguments in favour of the study of cellular senescence (see, for instance, *Strehler,* 1967, and *von Hahn,* 1971). It may, for instance, be noted that *Burnet* (1970, 1974) advocated the idea that if a single very important organ loses its capacity for cell proliferation this could be enough to release the phenomenon of senescence. He believes that ageing is characterized by autoimmune processes depending on a progressive weakening of immunological surveillance. *Burnet* believes that this weakening may be related to the degeneration of the thymus-dependent immune system.

b. Human Fibroblasts. Ageing Mutants

Using the technique of the culture of human fibroblasts, *Holliday and Tarrant* (1972) showed that diploid human fibroblasts accumulate heat-labile glucose-6-phosphate dehydrogenase during the final stages of their life-span in culture. Furthermore, cells grown for many generations in the presence of 5-fluorouracil, which induces errors in protein synthesis, become prematurely senescent. The premature senescence is accompanied by the appearance of a significant fraction of heat-labile glucose-6-phosphate dehydrogenase. It must be noted that these results have not been confirmed. *Pendergrass et al.* (1975) cultured *in vitro* a strain of diploid fibroblasts derived from skin. The cells were tested throughout their life-span for the appearance of altered glucose-6-phosphate dehydrogenase detected either by thermostability studies or by immunotitration. No significant difference was found in the proportion of the thermolabile enzyme in 31 young cultures in comparison with that in 19 old cultures.

In relation with premature senescence, a word must be said about the use of cell-cultures derived from so-called ageing mutants. The Hutchinson-Gilford syndrome or progeria and the Werner's syndrome are grave human diseases due to rare autosomal recessive mutations. The Down's syndrome is due to the trisomy of chromosome 21. These three genetic disorders obviously accelerate ageing, at least in some of its aspects and provoke a premature death. In each syndrome, however, there are abnormalities which are clearly unrelated to accelerated ageing, as well as an absence of many features which characterize normal ageing. Furthermore, those features which resemble to premature senescence are often quantitatively or qualitatively distinct from what is observed in the elderly (a review in *Tice and Schneider,* 1976).

The evidence concerning a variety of characteristics related to ageing and observed in cell cultures derived from patients suffering from progeria or Werner's syndrome is interesting but inconsistent and inconclusive. It was shown that fibroblasts obtained from patients suffering either from progeria (*Goldstein,* 1969) or from Werner's syndrome (*Martin et al.,* 1970) could only be subcultured *in vitro* for a very limited number of cell generations and this was very significantly less than the average life-span *in vitro* of fibroblasts from normal individuals of the same age. However, approximately normal life-spans of progeria fibroblasts *in vitro* have also been reported (*Martin et al.,* 1970; *Danes,*

1971). We have seen that during the rapid and premature ageing of progeria fibroblasts, these *in vitro* cell cultures show a concomitant decrease in activity of the DNA repair enzyme system (*Epstein et al.,* 1973). We did also note the conflicting results of *Epstein et al.* (1973) and of *Regan and Setlow* (1974). At present, it is not known if such contradistinctions should be attributed to a genetic heterogeneity of the patients tested or to differences in cell culture techniques.

Anyhow, it was shown that the changes which occurred in the glucose-6-phosphate dehydrogenase during the senescence of normal fibroblasts also occurred during the premature senescence of cells from a patient with Werner's syndrome (*Holliday et al.,* 1974). This series of observations does of course neither contradict nor verify the Orgel's 'error-catastrophe theory of ageing'.

Indeed, to deduce what ageing is from the analysis of phenomena which occur in lethal or sublethal mutants may appear dangerous. The same criticism may be made of another interesting experiment. In *Neurospora crassa,* a mutant called leu-5 produced an altered enzyme, leucyl-tRNA synthetase, which is believed to induce at 35 °C the incorporation into proteins of a series of amino acids in the place of leucine. When such a mutant is grown at 35 °C, it can be seen by analysis of the glutamine dehydrogenase, that a high proportion of altered molecules accumulate during the final stages of the culture (*Lewis and Holliday,* 1970). This shows that a lethal protein error-catastrophe may occur. However, the initial reason for that catastrophe being a mutation, this does not demonstrate that 'normal' ageing is due to an error-catastrophe.

Recently, *Holliday* and co-workers brooded over an enzyme which certainly plays a paramount role during the macromolecular synthesis of dividing cells, namely DNA polymerase (*Linn et al.,* 1976). They compared its activity in late versus early passage cells of the diploid human fibroblast line MRC-5. The level of activity dropped with increasing passage. In addition, when the fidelity of polymerization was monitored with four synthetic templates under a variety of conditions, it was observed that the enzyme from late passage cells was more error-prone. In accordance with Orgel's theory, the appearance and accumulation of error-prone DNA polymerase would be due to mistakes in transcription, translation or protein processing. In addition, the altered DNA polymerase molecules would themselves play a crucial role by introducing a high-frequency of genetic errors. Of course, an alternative possibility, which did not escape the authors, is that a new and error-prone DNA polymerase appears prior to ageing that has the specific function of causing cellular senescence.

2. Cons
Some minor objections to Orgel's hypothesis have recently been raised by *Baird et al.* (1975). The essence of their argument rests on the data gathered by *Finch* (1972) and *Wilson* (1973) which show that the activity of most enzymes

either remains unchanged or rises in senescent rodents. Clearly, this is not incompatible with Orgel's hypothesis, since a small number of errors in a few enzymes could be enough to kill a cell or an organism. At the present time, who can estimate the number of such errors and the number and type of such enzymes? Furthermore, and this point has been raised by the objectors to the error-catastrophe theory, if one admits that ageing and death are programmed, sequential and organized phenomena, then the increase, stability or decrease in the activity of an enzyme does not constitute an argument either in favour or against the error-catastrophe theory; indeed, those variations or absence of modifications may simply be considered as programmed. In addition, as was correctly stressed by *Holliday* (1975), Orgel's theory does not predict that the specific activity of an enzyme will show a significant decline with age. There may be a decline which is too small to measure, or even an increase in specific activity if regulatory mechanisms are affected.

Finally, it may be noted that the error-catastrophe theory does not predict the rate at which errors in macromolecular synthesis will accumulate and provoke cellular death. A progressive accumulation of erroneous macromolecules may be cataclysmic and, therefore, escape any experimental detection. Consequently, the absence of experimental detection in ageing cells of faulty macromolecules, bad-functioning enzymes, wrongly coded nucleic acids, and so on, does absolutely *not* constitute a demonstration of the falseness of the theory. A direct refutation of Orgel's theory by means either of an absence of erroneous molecules or by evidence showing the smooth working of the coding and/or decoding machinery of ageing cells appears to be really impossible. Such negative or positive evidence would at most restrict the application field of the theory to cellular death and no more to the entirety of the manifestations of ageing and senescence.

In the same way, it must be stressed that it is apparently also difficult to give a direct proof of the justness of Orgel's random theory. Indeed, one may easily conceive a developmental senescence mediated through the programmed appearance of slightly transformed macromolecules or even of new nonsense macromolecules whose role is to provoke a chain of deteriorative changes. In other words: the catastrophe could be programmed.

Thus, arguments against the error-catastrophe theory cannot be of a direct nature. An eventual refutation of the theory must rather depend on indirect evidence. In other words: Are there one or more biological phenomena related to development, differentiation, ageing and senescence which may not be understood in the light of the error-catastrophe theory?

a. Viruses

There are recent experiments by *Holland et al.* (1973) which, in relation to Orgel's theory, will perhaps appear one day as important as the experiments of

Clark and Rubin (1961) are for the mutation theory. *Holland* and his colleagues followed a simple reasoning. If ageing human fibroblasts, W1-38 human fibroblasts in phase III, i.e. after 50–60 passages synthesize much abnormal proteins, then replication and maturation of viruses in such aged fibroblasts should be affected. They therefore infected young and aged cells by different types of viruses – vesicular stomatitis virus, type 1 poliovirus and herpes simplex virus type 1 – and counted the yield. The experimental answer was extremely clear: the yield per cell was identical in young and in ageing cells. Not only was the quantity equal but also the quality of the collected viruses. This was shown by measuring, at 55 °C, the rate of inactivation of the infectivity of the produced virions which was seen to be identical in both types of virus. This was further confirmed by the comparison of the rate of mutations to guanidine resistance of polioviruses grown in senescent or low passage cells: the rates were identical.

These results have been confirmed and specified by several authors. Working with polio- and herpesvirus, *Tomkins* and his colleagues analyzed the quantity of virus produced, the pattern of cytopathology, the plaque morphology and the herpesvirus proteins in virus progeny produced in young or old W1-38 cells. They did not observe any significant difference (*Tomkins et al.,* 1974). In the same way, *Pitha et al.* (1974) studied infection by vesicular stomatitis virus in cultured human fibroblast cells of the W1-38 strain of varying senescence levels. They showed that, except during the last passage before the death by senescence of the W1-38 cell strain, the vesicular stomatitis virus replicated at the same rate.

These data seem to be incompatible with a generalized translation error-catastrophe theory. More complex hypotheses may be proposed. A restricted translational error catastrophe could occur through errors in some unusual codons. Viruses may have evolved in such a way to be able to replicate and mature in spite of translational errors.

One of the implications of that last hypothesis was tested by *Pitha et al.* (1975) and shown to be wrong. They supposed that late passage cells may synthesize viral proteins which contain sequence errors but are subsequently eliminated during virion formation. They used poliovirus to infect a W1-38 cell strain. It is known that the single poliovirus mRNA is translated into a single precursor protein which is then gradually cleaved into a series of smaller viral proteins. It is also known (*Jacobson et al.,* 1970) that when a permanent cell line as HeLa is infected by poliovirus and treated by amino acid analogues, the large precursor viral proteins, which presumably contain sequence errors, are left unprocessed in the cell. The authors therefore reasoned that the insertion – due to the senescence of the cells – of an incorrect amino acid into the precursor would produce an effect similar to the insertion of an analogue. By analyzing the various subgroups of newly synthesized proteins in W1-38 cells at different passages, they were able to show that no significant accumulation of large molecular weight proteins occurred in late passage cells compared with early ones.

Recently, *Fulder* (1977) used three temperature-sensitive mutants of *herpes* virus to infect human fibroblasts of the MRC-5 strain and looked at the reversion frequency in virus harvested from young and old cells. His results are extremely ambiguous, but show that in testing the error-catastrophe theory viral probes could be of a limited use. He found that with one of the temperature-sensitive mutants tested there was a 40-fold increase in reversion rate in the old cells compared to the young; with another, the rates were roughly similar and, with the third, a 100-fold decrease was observed in old cells! It was also shown that these differences were not due to differential rates of virus production.

It is possible that virus production in infected cells is insensitive to a number of distortions which may exist as well in young as in old cells and which, eventually, may be of importance for the survival of the cells. One should know if errors introduced artificially in the translational machinery of a cell result in two parallel effects, namely a rapid senescence and death of the cell *and* the production of altered virions.

b. *In vivo* Observations

We stressed the absence of obvious relations between the ageing of an organism and the senescence of a cell strain. In other words, there is at the moment no definite proof that the study of the phenomena linked to the ageing which happen in a cell culture bear to the actual senescence of the species from which the cells are issued. Therefore, one may guess that *in vivo* observations are and will be of a paramount importance in solving the problem of ageing. *In vivo* observations on a variety of species are obviously more difficult to achieve than *in vitro* observations on cell cultures.

We will first review some experiments which were made to test directly one of the implications of the error-catastrophe theory, namely the pernicious influence on life-span of the incorporation of amino acid analogues into the proteins of a living organism. Secondly, we will see to what extent the observations made on the enzymatic proteins of an organism at various moments of its life cycle do or do not confirm the predictions of the theory. It is, however, clear that the very best way to understand how *in vitro* and *in vivo* ageing are related and determined would be through the *concomitant* observations of *in vivo* and *in vitro* senescence and death. This may appear to be an impossible task. It is certainly not an easy task, but some few observations of that type have been made. They will be discussed in a later chapter (p. 57).

Harrison and Holliday (1967) experimentally tested the error-catastrophe theory by feeding various amino acid analogues to third instar larvae of *D. melanogaster* (fig. 8). They observed a decrease in life-span of the emerged imagos (p. 26). This confirms, at first view, one of the predictions of the error-catastrophe theory: agents which are expected to increase the number of errors in protein synthesis shorten life-span. Two other hypotheses may,

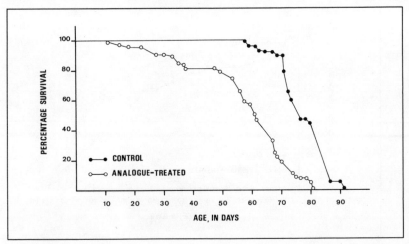

Fig. 8. Survival curve of hybrid F_1 males of *D. melanogaster* treated, as third instar larvae, for 24 h by various amino acid analogues (ethionine, *p*-fluorophenylalanine, canavanine, β2-thienylalanine and 4-methyl tryptophan). The mean imaginal life-span of the treated flies is significantly lower than the control. Redrawn with permission from *Harrison and Holliday* (1967).

however, be made — and were made by the authors. One may assume that amino acid analogues are, prior to metamorphosis, incorporated in proteins which last throughout the life of the adult flies. One knows indeed that about 80% of the proteins of *Drosophila* adults do not turn over during adult life and that only 20% turn over with a half-life approximately equal to 10 days (*Clarke and Maynard Smith*, 1966; *Maynard Smith et al.*, 1970). Such proteins with incorporated amino acid analogues could be functionally defective and, therefore, shorten life-span not because of an accumulation of defective and newly synthesized molecules, but simply because of a lowering of the metabolic efficiency. One could also assume that the toxicity of the treatment with amino acid analogues destroys or gravely damages, just prior to or during metamorphosis, a certain number of cells. This could produce some relatively non-visible morphological abnormalities which may shorten life-span.

With a view to distinguish between these two possibilities and Orgel's hypothesis, *Dingley and Maynard Smith* (1969) fed various amino acid analogues, but principally *p*-fluorophenylalanine (*p*-FPA), to young *adult* male *D. subobscura* and measured their effects on subsequent longevity of the flies surviving the treatment. A decrease in longevity in such an experiment would of course strongly confirm the error-catastrophe theory. They have first shown that *p*-FPA is effectively incorporated into the proteins of adult flies. Secondly, they

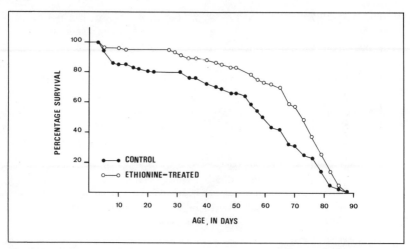

Fig. 9. Survival curves of Oregon wild-type males of *D. melanogaster* treated, as newly emerged imagos, for 72 h by ethionine, the analogue of methionine. In the experiment represented by the figure, the mean life-span of the treated flies equals 66.5 ± 2.0 days, whilst it equals 52.6 ± 3.5 days for the control flies, a significant difference at the 0.002 level. In two other experiments (not shown here), there are *no* significant differences between the treated and control flies. Redrawn with permission from *Bozcuk* (1976).

showed that flies kept continuously on *p*-FPA die almost as quickly as flies in which almost all protein synthesis has been stopped by a treatment with cycloheximide (*Dingley and Maynard Smith,* 1968). From this, it may be deduced that *p*-FPA adversely affects the functioning of several enzymes. Therefore, if errors in protein synthesis may provoke a catastrophe, then the treatment with *p*-FPA must be expected to shorten life-span. Yet feeding sub-lethal doses of *p*-FPA to young adults produces *no* shortening of life. (In fact, in one experiment a small increase in life-span of the treated flies was observed.) This makes it unlikely that the mechanism suggested by the error-catastrophe theory is an important cause of ageing in *Drosophila.* These results have been fully confirmed by *Bozcuk* (1976) working with *D. melanogaster* adult males (fig. 9).

Research conducted on cell cultures *in vitro,* as may be seen from the data reviewed above, recently became quite popular among gerontologists. However, as we have seen, the loss of capacity for division of a cell culture *in vitro* may have little to do with the *in vivo* causes of ageing, simply because it is unlikely that animals age because one or more important cell populations lose their proliferative capacity. Furthermore, even if Orgel's catastrophes occur in single cells of *in vitro* cultures this does not, of couse, demonstrate that the same occurs *in vivo.* And, even if they do occur *in vivo,* cellular redundancy, as pointed out by *Burch and Jackson* (1976), may render negligible the consequences of such chain errors. A series of experiments, mainly by the *Gershons,* throw some light on that problem.

If the error-catastrophe theory of ageing is correct, reasoned the *Gershons,* altered protein molecules should appear in ageing organisms in quantities which are direct function of increasing age. In other words, the enzyme molecules of aged organisms should show reduced catalytic activity. The activity must of course be calculated either per unit weight of the purified protein or per antigenic unit of the enzyme. They were indeed able to show, both in nematodes and in rodents, that there was an age-related accumulation of antigenically cross-reacting material either devoid of, or with reduced catalytic activity. In the nematode *Turbatrix aceti,* the specific activity of isocitrate lyase (*Gershon and Gershon,* 1970) and of fructose 1,6-diphosphate aldolase (*Zeelon et al.,* 1973) was shown to decrease with advancing age. In *Mus musculus,* the specific activity of liver fructose 1,6-diphosphate aldolase was shown to decrease as a function of age (*Gershon and Gershon,* 1973a). In the same organism, the specific activity of muscle aldolase was found to be invariable with age although the quantity of aldolase in old mice was 1.3–1.4 times higher than in young mice; this implies that, in older animals, many aldolase molecules are inactive (*Gershon and Gershon,* 1973b). Interestingly enough, no obvious catastrophic increase in erroneous proteins has ever been observed either in nematodes or in mice. In other words, the increase and accumulation of cross-reacting material appear to be gradual throughout the life-span of the organism and, furthermore, this appears to start at a relatively young age. These results have recently been confirmed in a number of laboratories (review in *Gershon and Gershon,* 1976).

The presence of altered protein molecules in old organisms is, of course, not enough to demonstrate the correctness of the error catastrophe theory. The altered proteins must be the results of faulty protein synthesis, i.e. of erroneous and stochastic misincorporation of amino acids during the synthesis of new proteins by old organisms. Therefore, for any specific enzyme, the population of molecules found in an old or in a senescent organism should range in catalytic activity from completely active through various degrees of partially active to totally inactive forms. For the time being, there is no direct evidence concerning the amino acid sequence of altered enzyme molecules in old organisms. However, indirect evidence abounds. Following *Gershon and Gershon* (1976), it has been shown, for a variety of enzymes, both in nematodes and in mice, that the electrophoretic mobility of the *active* enzyme, the antigenic identity, the affinity for substrate and for specific inhibitors, and the molecular weight are unchanged as a function of age (*Gershon and Gershon,* 1970, 1973a, b; *Zeelon et al.,* 1973; *Gershon et al.,* 1974; *Reiss and Rothstein,* 1974, 1975; *Bollo and Brot,* 1975). *Active* enzyme molecules in ageing organisms are thus indistinguishable from those present in young organisms. Therefore, the cross-reacting material undoubtedly present in old animals must be composed *only* of totally inactive molecules. Although, surprisingly enough, these data have been considered as an argument in favour of Orgel's hypothesis (*Baird et al.*, 1975), they constitute in fact a clear negation of the 'error-catastrophe theory which predicts random errors in protein synthesis which then lead to infidelity and should produce enzyme molecules with a whole spectrum of activities' (*Gershon and Gershon*, 1976).

c. Transformation – Totipotency

The analysis of cell cultures not only yields results concerning age-related biochemical variations in senescent cells but, through the study of the phenomenon of transformation, also throws some light on the control mechanisms of cell multiplication, differentiation and survival.

Transformation exists both in animal cells in culture and in plant cells. This phenomenon exhibits some interesting features obviously related to ageing. Although there is no single reliable and generally accepted criterion to define transformation, and although it is impossible to define accurately what a normal, a transformed or a reverted cell is, it may very broadly be said that transformation in animal cells is correlated with a loss of growth control as well *in vivo,* as shown by the induction of various types of malignancy, as *in vitro,* as shown by their ability to multiply in conditions that inhibit the multiplication of normal cells. Another characteristic of the transformed cells which is directly related to the present topic is their unlimited life-span in cultures. Without entering into all the characteristics, some of which are disputed, that have been ascribed to these various types of cells, it is interesting to note that the passage both of a normal cell strain with limited life-span to a transformed 'eternal' cell line, and of a transformed cell line to a reverted cell strain with limited life-span, are accompanied by variations in the genetic information content as demonstrated by the heritable state of both transformed and reverted states. It is therefore obvious that the expression of transformation – as measured by malignancy or life-span of cell lines – may be modulated or suppressed.

Various treatments, by viruses, chemical carcinogens and so on, may transform mammalian cells in culture from a mortal to an immortal state. Such transformation may also occur spontaneously. The relation between the error-catastrophe theory and transformation is not obvious! More precisely, it is not clear how a transforming treatment may render protein synthesis more precise. However, it has been suggested (*Orgel,* 1973) that an increased mitotic rate or some other mechanism could give to such transformed cells a better protection against the accumulation of errors. *Ryan et al.* (1974) have tested this idea by measuring the sensitivity to a wide range of concentrations of amino acid analogues of a permanent cell line on the one side – human cells transformed by simian virus 40 (SV40) — and of a normal diploid W1-38 human cell strain on the other side. At all concentrations, the two cell cultures show similar sensitivities.

Transformation does not appear to be a random phenomenon. On the contrary, it exhibits some interesting features which point clearly to the fact that the phenomenon is to some extent genetically controlled. This has of course implications directly relevant to the problem under discussion, i.e. the relation between genetics and ageing. If it could be demonstrated that transformation is genetically controlled, then there would be some ground to admit that the various manifestations linked to it are also under genetic control.

Rabinowitz and Sachs studied in hamster embryo cell cultures the properties of normal, transformed and reverted cells — more specifically their finite or infinite life-span in culture, and their malignancy. Using various carcinogens, namely polyoma and the chemical dimethylnitrosamine, they were able to induce the formation of cultures with an infinite life-span. A reversion to finite life-span was afterwards obtained in a certain number of cases (*Rabinowitz and Sachs*, 1970a, 1972). They claimed that the expression and suppression of transformed properties were presumably dependent on a balance between factors responsible for expression — E factors — and their suppressors — S factors. They have assumed that the E factors present in a normal cell are neutralized by S factors. Different agents may then modify the balance between E and S factors, leading the cell to a transformed and, eventually, a reverted state (*Rabinowitz and Sachs*, 1970b). Later on, they studied the karyotypes of various types of normal, transformed and reverted cells and showed that the passage from one stage to another was clearly linked to a change — either a decrease or an increase — in the number of chromosomes (*Hitotsumachi et al.*, 1971). More recently, using the Giemsa technique to identify individual chromosomes, they claimed the E genes to be located in the 5_7 and 5_{10} chromosomes, and the S genes in the 7_3 and 7_{10} chromosomes (*Yamamoto et al.*, 1973).

In mouse tumour cell cultures, malignancy can be suppressed when malignant cells are fused with non-malignant ones. Malignancy thus appears as a recessive character. Reversion to malignancy in the segregating progeny of the fused cells is associated with a loss of specific chromosomes (*Harris et al.*, 1969). These chromosomes are as yet unidentified. Complementation analysis after fusion between various tumorous cells generated only one clone with a reduced tumorigenicity among 42 clonal populations studied; in all other cases, the hybrid cells formed were highly malignant. If non-complementation has the same biological significance both in differentiated somatic cells and in other organisms, then the authors are faced with the conclusion, which for obvious reasons they consider with great reserve, that malignancy, at least in a wide range of these mice tumour cells, is determined by a recessive at a single locus (*Wiener et al.*, 1974).

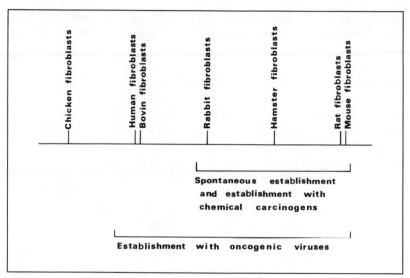

Fig. 10. Fibroblasts from different animal species do not have identical probabilities of yielding cell lines with an unlimited growth potential, either spontaneously or under the influence of chemical carcinogens. The probability is low for chicken fibroblasts; at the other end of the scale, mice fibroblasts invariably originate spontaneous permanent cell lines when explanted *in vitro*. Redrawn with permission from *Macieira-Coelho et al.* (1977).

Macieira-Coelho et al. (1977) gathered impressive evidence related to the life-span of fibroblast cultures. They have shown that there are good reasons to believe that the limited or unlimited life-span of cultivated fibroblasts is related to the animal species. In fact, when one compares the fibroblasts from different species in regard to the probability of yielding lines with an unlimited growth potential, one finds a gradient-like pattern extending from cultures which invariably die after a certain number of passages to other cultures which invariably acquire an infinite division potential (fig. 10). For instance, chicken fibroblasts never give rise to a permanent cell line either spontaneously or after treatment with chemicals (*Ponten*, 1971). They can give rise to permanent cell lines only if kept at 40 °C after infection with oncogenic viruses (*Macieira-Coelho*, personal communication). On the contrary, and on the opposite end of the scale, mouse fibroblast cultures invariably originate permanent cell lines spontaneously (*Todaro and Green*, 1963). The case of human fibroblasts is intermediate. Human fibroblasts, as we have seen, have a limited life-span *in vitro*. They may, however, be transformed into permanent cell lines after infection with the oncogenic virus SV40 (*Girardi et al.*, 1965) and other DNA viruses. They do not originate spontaneously permanent cell lines. Nor are they transformed by chemical

carcinogens, with one exception which is of great interest. Human skin fibroblasts treated *in vitro* with urethane yielded two permanent cell lines; the cells
were obtained from siblings suffering from the von Recklinghausen's syndrome,
a familial disorder characterized by multiple fibromas with a high predisposition
to malignant transformation *in vivo.* The von Recklinghausen's syndrome is
controlled by a dominant autosomal gene (*Benedict et al.,* 1975). This does of
course not demonstrate that for human fibroblasts the property to acquire a
transformed state and more specifically an infinite life-span is determined by the
autosomal dominant gene responsible for the von Recklinghausen's syndrome,
but suggests that that property is under genetic control.

It always appeared strange to me that scientists working with animal cell
cultures ignore the work of their colleagues on plant cell cultures. And vice
versa, of course! Vegetal cell cultures are really magnificent material. One should
bear in mind that the first demonstration of cell totipotency was obtained from
a phloem culture of *Daucus carotta* (*Steward et al.,* 1958a, b; a review of the
earlier more or less successful attempts in *Steward,* 1968). However, as far as we
know, no finite life-span of vegetal cells in culture has ever been noticed. They
can grow and multiply for years. *Torrey* (1967) has reported of callus tissues of
root tips of *Pisum sativum* grown successfully for more than 10 years, and
periodically tested for their capacity to initiate roots. It was shown that during
that long period of culture there was a progressive loss of organ-forming capacity
which was paralleled by an increasing number of abnormalities in the chromosomal constitution, including higher chromosome numbers and higher frequency
of aneuploidy. One may, *mutatis mutandis,* compare these abnormal vegetal
cells, just able to grow and to divide, with transformed animal cells.

In *D. carotta,* the transition from the proliferated, comparatively regular but
unorganized growth of explanted pieces of phloem tissue to the development of
cell colonies which achieve a level of organization permitting the development of
whole plants goes through a stage of growth of completely free and rather
diversified cells (*Steward et al.,* 1958a, b). *Mitra et al.* (1960) examined the
nuclei and chromosomes of cells at various stages, namely during the growth of a
tissue culture from an explant of secondary phloem, during the growth and
multiplication of free cells in a liquid medium and during growth and reforma-
tion of roots or whole plants. *D. carotta* has a diploid cell number of 18.
Interestingly enough, the cells which develop in the explant and the cells of the
reformed organs, including the flowers — where normal meiosis occurs (*Steward
et al.,* 1961) — are also diploid. On the contrary, the free cells are characterized
by a wide range and 'a rich diversity' of cytological aberrations: tetraploidy, high
polyploidy, haploidy, chromosomal abnormalities and so on.

This series of evidence shows that a cell may pass from a more or less
anarchic to an organized condition. The most important function of a cell in a
state of anarchy is to reproduce, and such reproduction may proceed *ad*

aeternum. The organized state has an essential consequence for the cell: the daughter cells produced by such a cell are essentially different from the mother cell. This is an inescapable conclusion which emerges from the fact that after a certain number of divisions the daughter cells will inevitably enter the ageing pathway, senesce and eventually die. The passage from non-organization to organization requires, of course, a complete and balanced genetic information but also a supplementary information provided by cellular interaction, and may be mediated through the action of morphogens as it was suggested by *Crick* (1970) (p. 89). Thus, far from appearing as a random phenomenon, 'reprogrammation' appears as a precise restoration of an orderly gene expression mediated through the action of gene-controlling molecules. The following two examples may be sufficient to illustrate that point.

It has been known since a certain time that embryonic tissues can influence tumours to undergo differentiation. A recent study, and probably the most complete, has shown that a murine mammary tumour will differentiate ducts if cultured *in vitro* with embryonic mouse mammary mesenchyme. Other types of cytodifferentiation, as delineated by histological evidence and histological staining techniques, are obtained when the tumour is grown *in vitro* with various other embryonic tissues. Furthermore, evidence for cytodifferentiation was also obtained after exposure of the tumour to the inductive tissues across a thin Millipore filter. The filter certainly excluded the passage of cells but possibly allowed direct contact of cell processes intruding from either side (*Decosse et al.*, 1975).

That in some cases malignancy in all likelihood does not involve mutational events results from some elegant experiments (fig. 11) which demonstrate unequivocally that mouse malignant teratocarcinoma cells are totipotent (*Mintz and Illmensee*, 1975; *Illmensee and Mintz,* 1976). In a first experiment, mouse teratocarcinoma *cells* bearing a genetic marker and with a normal modal chromosome number were taken from the cores of embryoid bodies grown exclusively *in vivo* for 8 years, and were injected into blastocysts bearing many genetic markers. The injected blastocysts were surgically transferred to the uteri of the pseudopregnant mice. A certain number of living animals were obtained. In one particular case, cells derived from the carcinoma were shown to have contributed to the germ line of one of these animals and to have formed reproductively functional sperms, some of which transmitted to the progeny the marker gene of the tumour cells (*Mintz and Illmensee,* 1975).

In a second experiment, a conclusive test for developmental totipotency of mouse malignant teratocarcinoma cells was conducted by cloning *singly injected cells* in genetically marked blastocysts. Totipotency was clearly shown in an adult mosaic female whose tumour-strain cells had made substantial contributions to all of its somatic tissues analyzed. Thus, embryonic body core cells appear to be developmentally totipotent after almost 200 transplant generations

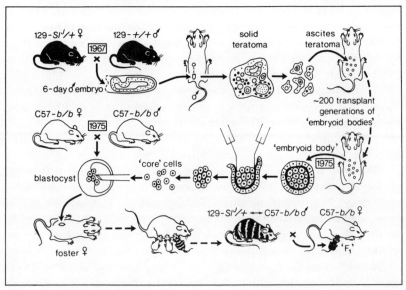

Fig. 11. Diagram of the experiments showing the totipotency and normal differentiation of single teratocarcinoma cells cloned by injection into mouse blastocysts. In a first experiment (the present diagram), *five* malignant core cells were injected into blastocysts later on transferred to pseudopregnant females. From the mice born a mosaic male was test-mated to genetically marked females. The production of F_1-like offspring proved that this male had normal sperms derived from the teratocarcinoma cells. In a later experiment, the same procedure was used throughout except that a *single* core cell was injected into the blastocysts. From *Mintz and Illmensee* (1975).

as a highly malignant tumour. They are indeed able to express many genes hitherto silent in the tumour of origin in an orderly sequence of differentiation of the somatic and germ line. This is an unequivocal example of a non-mutational basis for transformation to malignancy and of reversal to normality (*Illmensee and Mintz*, 1976).

The comparison between animal and vegetal cell cultures may apparently lead to one generalization, namely that an unlimited potential to grow and to divide is accompanied by more or less important chromosomal abnormalities, going from simple insertion into the chromosomes of the genetic information of an oncogenic virus to gross chromosomal aberrations involving various forms of poly- or aneuploidy. The size, the shape, the nuclear behaviour, the affinity, the morphogenetic relationships with other cells, and so on are drastically modified. The more a cell forgets apparently what it is supposed to do, the more it appears unbalanced; the more it is *deprogrammed,* the more it will divide and live. The transition from a normal cell with finite life-span to an abnormal cell with infinite life-span involves modifications of cellular regulation events which may stem from changes in the genome, as a result of somatic mutations or induction by carcinogens or oncogenic viruses. This is not a new idea; it was first suggested by *Boveri* as early as 1914 when he proposed that the expression of malignancy could originate from chromosomal imbalance.

This represents in fact the classical idea favoured by some oncologists, who assume that a modification of the genetic information of a differentiated cell results in a process of dedifferentiation, the overt manifestations of which are a neoplastic cellular state, a more or less anarchic multiplication and phenotypic traits different from those of a normal tissue.

This view is not universally accepted. Some authors accept that mutations, in the broadest sense of the word, may in some cases be responsible for malignancy, but suggest an alternative explanation. They assume that malignancy may be due to changes in the cytoplasmic components, stimulated by one or the other carcinogen and which would alter the *control* of the nuclear function and lead to a massive new read-off of some part of the genetic information normally repressed (*Pierce,* 1970; *Pierce and Johnson,* 1971). We guess it is only in the light of that hypothesis that reversion and the drastic modifications in behaviour which accompany it may be understood. From that point of view, transformation *and* reversion, cytodifferentiation of tumour cells, totipotency and more specifically totipotency and normal differentiation of tumour cells, which are all unaccountable in terms of the error-catastrophe theory, become perfectly understandable.

D. The Developmental Theory of Ageing

Muller (1963) has argued that development is a continuous process of which senescence forms the last stage or, in other words, that ageing is a built-in consequence of differentiation. From a review of the mechanisms of life-span shortening, he concluded, 'that spontaneous ageing is a part of normal development caused, like most other developmental changes, by other factors than permanent genetic alterations such as point-mutation, deficiency, chromosome loss or inactivation, or segregation, even though it does involve the point-wise death of many individual somatic cells'.

Comfort (1968) noticed that if ageing is a consequence of differentiation caused, for instance, by the switching-off of synthetic processes which cannot be switched on again without loss of differentiation or to the evolutionary accumulation of late-acting deleterious genes, such an implication has at least one important consequence, namely that the only likely way of prolonging vigour would come through a stretching of the developmental programme as a whole and essentially, according to *Comfort,* through a prolongation of immaturity.

Such a statement is most probably correct (a prolongation of life through a prolongation of the maturity is not entirely unknown), but could also be incomplete. Indeed, that statement, which links senescence to differentiation, implies that senescence is genetically determined. This may mean that development and ageing are directed by totally different sets of genes; it may also mean that senescence and some aspects of development are controlled by an identical information or by an identical chain of information. In the last hypothesis, a genetic or environmental interference with that or those particular aspects of development must be reflected in variations of the time of onset of ageing and/or in variations of life-span. The relevant evidence must be considered *in vivo* at the level both of the organism and of the cell.

1. The Relation between Growth and Ageing
a. Homeotherms

McCay et al. (1935, 1939) are generally credited as being the first to have shown that retarded growth of the albino rat, provoked by a deficiency in the daily allowance of energy in the diet, resulted in a longer life-span. They showed indeed that when growth was retarded for 300, 500, 700 or 1,000 days, the mean life-span could be prolonged by 150–300 days roughly. However, the period of adult life tends to be shorter after long retardation; in fact, the part of life remaining after maturation is a negative function of the length of the retarded period (table XI). In earlier days, *Osborne and Mendel* (1915, 1916) and *Osborne et al.* (1917) had shown essentially the same thing on a smaller sample of rats.

Table XI. Life-span of female and male albino rats maintained for different periods of time under a highly restricted diet. The diet given to the restricted animals was determined by the amount needed to maintain the retarded animals at an almost stationary weight. After different periods of time, the restricted animals were fed in such a way as to reach maturity. The mean life-span of the control group (n = 33) equals 657 ± 27 days

Length of restricted diet regimen days	Mean life-span days	Mean time lived after growth completion days	Number of animals observed
300	835 ± 68	535	9
500	898 ± 71	457	9
700	896 ± 80	253	10
1,000	949 ± 95	138	9

Recalculated from tables 3 and 4 in *McCay et al.* (1939).

These results have been extended to various other species, both in invertebrates and in vertebrates (review in *Silberberg and Silberberg,* 1955); they have been specified, at least to a certain extent, as to the respective parts played by proteins, carbohydrates and lipids (review in *Silberberg and Silberberg,* 1955; *Ross,* 1959). Modifications in the dietary habits of young or even adult animals modify the expectation of life. The following generalization may be done without any great risk of error: underfeeding increases the length of life, whilst overfeeding or other dietary excess or unbalance decreases it. Although interesting insofar as they show that a modification of the metabolic rate may influence adult life-span, these links between diet and ageing do not solve the problem of determinism – genetic or environmental? – of the relation between growth rate and longevity. In fact, they only do show that when the metabolic activity of an individual is too high and when the organism is too much solicited the duration of life is reduced. These effects may thus be considered as being almost entirely of a mechanical nature; the higher the wear and tear, the lower the expectation of life.

More interesting, in the present respect, are the studies which look at the modification in life-span brought about by selection for various components of growth or linked to the natural variation of these components which may exist in a given population.

Roberts (1961) studied the life-span of four strains of mice, two of them selected for a high 6-week weight, i.e. for a fast growth rate, and two others selected for a low 6-week weight, i.e. for a slow growth rate. The comparison between fast- and slow-growing mice shows that the slow-growing are longer-lived than the fast-growing (table XII). The average length of life over all stocks was 1 year and 8 months; the mean life-span of the slow-growing strains exceeded that of the fast-growing by approximately 6 months. Furthermore, the large strains had a short reproductive life, producing on average only 4.5 litters, against eleven or so in the small strains. On account of this, the small strains eventually weaned almost twice as many offspring as the large strains. Other differences – related to the variation of weight during life-time, number of offspring per litter, and so on – were also observed.

Two conclusions emerge from that study. Firstly, the selection for a rapid early growth has an adverse effect on reproductive fitness, as judged by the total number of offspring weaned over life-time. This reduction in number of offspring resulted mainly from a drastic shortening of the length of reproductive life. Secondly, in general the correlated responses to selection found are in opposite direction in the fast- and in the slow-growing stocks. That last point is particularly important.

A natural population may be defined by a system of gene frequencies which, as a first approximation, may be considered to have been brought about by the effect of natural selection. The existing array of gene frequencies and

Table XII. Average life-span (in days) of various non-selected and selected groups of mice. RCL is a stock — issued from a cross between two strains of large mice — selected for high 6-week weight for ten generations. MS is a stock — issued from a small selected strain — selected for low 6-week weight for 17 generations. M × R is an hybrid F_1 stock, produced by crossing reciprocally the RCL and MS strains. NF was selected for high 6-week weight for 27 generations, NS for low 6-week weight for 22 generations. NC is an unselected control stock. Note that in the case of the N stocks, and unexpectedly, selection in either direction increased life-span

Strain	Male	Female
RCL (fast growth)	474 ± 32	284 ± 30
MS (slow growth)	700 ± 44	452 ± 53
M × R	683 ± 66	471 ± 60
NF (fast growth)	759 ± 63	731 ± 75
NS (slow growth)	900 ± 99	747 ± 73
NC	493 ± 79	545 ± 81

From *Roberts* (1961).

consequently the existing genetic properties of a population thus represent the best total adjustment to existing conditions that is possible with the available genetic variation. If a population is in genetic equilibrium, it follows that a reduction of fitness must in principle result from *any* changes in the array of gene frequencies, such as those eventually caused by selection in either direction. This principle is called genetic homeostasis (*Lerner,* 1954). In *Robert's* experiment, the correlated responses to selection found were usually in opposite directions in the fast- and slow-growing stocks. On the basis of a homeostatic model, this is of course not what is expected from characters related to fitness. Correlated response of two characters — in the present case growth rate and life-span — to selection for one of those characters cannot arise in the absence of a genetic correlation between those traits. A genetic correlation implies either that some genes affect both characters, i.e. are pleiotropic, or that genes affecting both characters are very closely linked (see *Falconer,* 1960, for a full discussion of the genetic correlation).

These results have been fully confirmed in a study of longevity and life-time body weight in mice selected for rapid growth (*Eklund and Bradford,* 1977). On the basis of the response to selection, rapid growth rate — as measured by the 3—6 weeks of age gain in weight — appears to be partly determined by the genotype and, importantly in the present respect, to be associated with a shortened life-span (fig. 12).

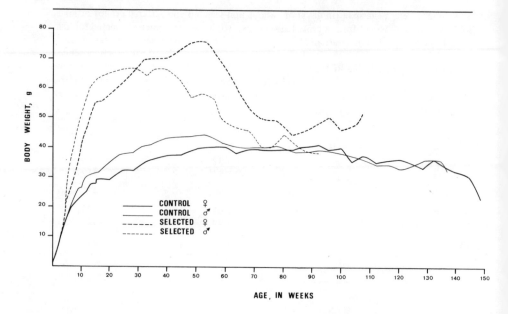

Fig. 12. Mean body weight as a function of time for female and male mice of a control unselected stock and of a strain selected for high body weight gain from 21 to 42 days of age. The mean life-span (in weeks) of these strains is: control ♀ 119.5 ± 3.2; control ♂ 112.1 ± 5.4; selected ♀ 82.3 ± 3.2; selected ♂ 51.1 ± 5.7. The number of animals observed equals 16 in each class. Redrawn from *Eklund and Bradford* (1977).

Dietary practices, specially during early life, and genetically determined growth rate have thus an influence on adult life-span of rodents. A study of *Ross et al.* (1976) has shown that several parameters which involve growth rate (table XIII) correlate more closely with life-span than any of the dietary variables (table XIV). The authors measured 16 variables related to dietary habits (daily food intake, protein intake, non-protein caloric intake, and so on) and growth rate (body weight at various fixed times, age to attain a specified weight, time to double weight, and so on) in a group of 120 rats. The animals were offered daily a choice of three different diets varying by the relative composition in protein and carbohydrate components. (Dietary preference of young animals may have a genetic basis.) The results show that regardless of the proximate cause of death there are combinations of specific conditions early in life which allow accurate prediction of individual life-span. More precisely: by the technique of the conditional multiple regression analysis (table XIII), the authors were able to estimate, by use of parameters related mainly to growth rate and

Table XIII. Correlation between life-span and variables related to growth rate in rats

Variable	Coefficient of correlation[1]	p
Weight gain[2]	− 0.44	<0.001
Maximum body weight attained	− 0.07	n.s.
Age to attain specified weight[3]	0.46	<0.001
Age-independent body weight acquisition time:		
For 100-gram increments[4]	0.48	<0.001
For body weight doubling[5]	0.49	<0.001

Modified from *Ross et al.* (1976).
[1] n = 120 or 121.
[2] Weight gain is computed for successive 7-week intervals.
[3] Age to attain specified weight is computed for successive 100-gram intervals between 300 and 600 g.
[4] From 200 to 300 g and from 500 to 600 g.
[5] From 200 to 400 g and from 300 to 600 g. All the significant correlations indicate that life-span is all the more longer as growth rate is slower.

accessorily to dietary practices, the individual life-span of the observed rats. In the words of the authors: 'The ability to make a long-range life-span forecast is all the more remarkable in that it incorporates differences in the age of onset and the rate of progression of one or more debilitating, fatal diseases.' One is in agreement with the authors in their conclusion that 'the individual specificity', the genotype which is responsible for the individual variations in growth rate, is also responsible for the onset of ageing and the time of death.

b. Poikilotherms

In homeotherms, a modification of the genetic information related to growth rate obtained by selection has thus important and coherent effects on life-span: the slower the growth rate, the longer the duration of life and vice versa. In the same way, the natural variations in growth rate appear to be correlated with the natural variations in life-span. Finally, a prolongation of total life-span, essentially through a serious prolongation of immaturity and probably at the sacrifice of a part of the adult longevity, may be obtained by various manipulations of the dietary habits, mainly during adolescence.

However, the question that may be asked is in how far the interference with the development and differentiation of an organism during adolescence does have any paramount effect on the future and latest steps of life. Indeed, at that stage of life, differentiation and development are for the most part completed. Interference during the earliest embryonic stages appears to be more promising.

Table XIV. Estimation by the conditional multiple regression analysis of the individual life-span of rats as determined from growth and dietary practices early in life. Dietary components are: gross food efficiency, protein intake and protein fraction of the diet or protein intake per kg body weight. Growth components are: body weight at 119 and 133 days, age at 500 g, body weight doubling time. The predictive capability of the multiple regression equation is improved parallel to the progressive elimination of the shortest-lived rats

Fraction of population %	Range in life-span days	Cohort size number	Estimated compared with actual life-span		Fraction of variance explained by			Contribution of growth factors, %
			correlation coefficient	absolute average error, %	growth and dietary factors	growth factors	dietary factors	
100	317–1,026	119	0.68	12.1	0.46	0.34	0.16	74
95	425–1,026	113	0.72	10.2	0.52	0.40	0.15	77
85	500–1,026	101	0.71	8.8	0.51	0.39	0.17	77
70	575–1,026	83	0.69	7.5	0.47	0.40	0.17	86
50	620–1,026	60	0.69	6.2	0.48	0.43	0.02	90
25	700–1,026	30	0.81	3.8	0.66	0.66	–	100

Modified from Ross et al. (1976).

In that respect, insects and other poikilotherms appear more suitable than homeotherms for use in testing a programmed senescence theory of ageing simply because their early developmental homeostatic mechanisms are not strictly regulated. We have manipulated the conditions – temperature and larval density – in which the pre-imaginal life of *D. melanogaster* is spent. In *D. melanogaster,* duration of development can be prolonged either by decreasing the temperature at which development occurs – six temperatures ranging from 31 to 16 °C were used – or by increasing the larval population density – eight different densities ranging from 3 to 480 eggs per standard vial. Decreasing the pre-imaginal temperature results in prolonged duration of development, larger adult size and a significant increase in imaginal life-span. Increasing the pre-imaginal population density results in prolonged duration of development, smaller size and a significant increase in life-span. Life-span is measured in standard conditions (fig. 13). An essential difference with *McCay*'s type of experiments must thus be stressed. The life-span measured in the *Drosophila* experiments is the time between imaginal emergence and death; it thus does *not* include the more or less extended period of time between fertilization and the emergence of the imago (*Lints and Lints,* 1969, 1971a, b). Correlations between life-span and the various quantitative traits related to growth and development – size, developmental time, growth rate – are then calculated. There is a highly significant negative correlation between growth rate – estimated as the ratio between the cube of the thoracic size and duration of development – and life-span. We explained our results by assuming that adult longevity is determined early in life by a defined programme. We further argued that this programme and growth rate could be concomitantly modified by varying the pre-imaginal environment (*Lints and Lints,* 1971c).

We believed that the above results and assumptions implied that within a species the variations in growth rate, characteristic of the various races of that species, should be reflected in the variations of life-spans of those races. In order to test this implication, we studied, in a single environment, the growth rate – measured as the larval weight at a fixed time – and life-span of eight wild strains of *Tribolium castaneum* of wide geographic origin. The variations in both traits are quite large and the relationship between them is positive and highly significant (fig. 13) (*Lints and Soliman,* 1977). It is worth emphasizing that the same study has shown that there is no strong correlation between life-span and development time or adult weight (*Soliman and Lints,* 1975).

Thus, in *Drosophila* an *artificially* obtained decrease in growth rate of a *single* hybrid genotype results in an increase in life-span while in *Tribolium* the *natural* variations in growth rate of *various* genotypes are positively correlated with life-span. Except for those differences in experimental approach, *Tribolium* and *Drosophila* differ at least in three major ways directly related to growth rate and ageing. Firstly, duration of development in *Tribolium* appears to be under

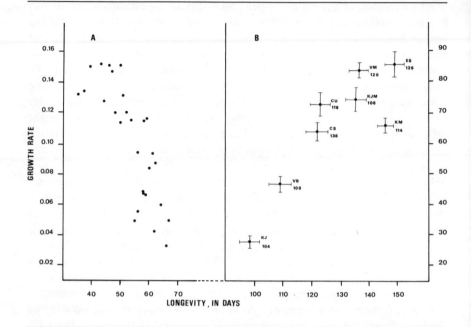

Fig. 13. A Adult longevity as a function of growth rate in *D. melanogaster* (r = − 0.801; n = 28; p <0.001). Growth rate is estimated as the ratio between the cube of the thoracic size and the duration of development. Longevity is measured at 25 °C on 14 samples of two reciprocal hybrids raised in various preimaginal environments − six different temperatures, eight different preimaginal population densities − which are known to modify both the size and the duration of development of the treated individuals. Redrawn from *Lints and Lints* (1971b). *B* Adult longevity ± standard error plotted against growth rate, measured as mean 13-day larval weight, of eight wild strains of *Tribolium castaneum*. The strains are identified according to their geographic origin as: CS (Capetown, South Africa), CU (Chicago, United States), ES (Edinburgh, Scotland), KJ (Kyoto, Japan), KJM (Kingston, Jamaica), KN (Kano, Nigeria), VB (Vicosa, Brazil) and VM (Veracruz, Mexico). Longevity measurement is based on observing adult death every 10 days up to a maximum of 227 days from egg. This period covered most of the adult death for all strains and the percentage of adults still alive after this period (with a maximum of 18% for ES) is highly correlated with the longevity estimates (r = 0.840; n = 8; p <0.01). Numbers indicate the sample size of each strain. Redrawn from *Lints and Soliman* (1977).

polygenic control (*Englert and Bell,* 1970), while selection for fast and slow development is generally unsuccessful in *Drosophila* (*Lints and Gruwez,* 1972). Secondly, the imaginal longevities of both species are quite different; in optimal conditions, the average longevity of *Drosophila* is about 50 days, while in *Tribolium* it is rather more than 130 days. Thirdly, contrary to *Drosophila*

(*Bozcuk*, 1972), somatic cell division occurs during the imaginal stages of the life cycle of *Tribolium* (*Devi et al.*, 1963).

In *Drosophila*, life-span thus appears to depend negatively on growth rate, which is the productivity of the genotype per unit of time that is the resultant of anabolism and catabolism due to genotype-environment interactions. Growth rate may be associated with mitotic division rate. When growth rate is accelerated or decelerated, it may, as a first approximation, be admitted that the same happens for mitotic division rate. *Bozcuk* (1972) has demonstrated that tissues of holometabolous insects, like *Drosophila*, show no mitoses after the emergence of the imago. The death of the organism must thus, to a certain extent, coincide with the cellular death. On the other hand, it is known from the studies carried out *in vivo* in higher organisms (for full details see *Bullough*, 1967) that, when a cell enters the ageing pathway, it has a life expectancy that is characteristic of the tissue. When the mitotic rate of the tissue is high, as in the intestinal lining, the life expectancy of the functional cell is only a few days (*Lesher et al.*, 1961); when the mitotic rate is moderate, as in epidermis, the life expectancy may be a few weeks (*van Scott and Ekel*, 1963); when the mitotic rate is low, as in liver, the life expectancy may exceed a year (*McDonald*, 1961). Furthermore, artificial prolongation of the epidermal cell life (*Bullough and Ebling*, 1952) and of the liver cell life (*McDonald*, 1961) was obtained in conditions of stress which provoked a decreased mitotic rate.

Those relations between growth rate, mitotic division rate and longevity do not unambiguously demonstrate the validity of the developmental theory of ageing, nor do they totally exclude the error-catastrophe theory. On the one hand, in relation with the developmental theory, it may be supposed – as was done to explain the influence of pre-imaginal temperature on adult life-span (*Burcombe and Hollingsworth*, 1970) – that the growth rate affects the type of molecules that are synthetized and the rate at which the molecules carry out metabolism. If the idea of morphogens (*Crick*, 1970) is accepted, it may then be supposed that variations in the type of molecules present in a cell affect the course of differentiation and development. Variations in the molecular composition of a cell as a function of growth rate are not unknown. (That point will be further discussed; p. 91.) A changing growth rate could thus result in a different cytoplasmic molecular composition or configuration which could explain an earlier or later programmed death of the cells and of the organism. But, on the other hand, in relation with the error-catastrophe theory, if a slower mitotic rate is accompanied by a lower number of errors of replication – a point which is not yet demonstrated – this could explain a later, randomly provoked, unprogrammed cellular and organismic death.

In *Tribolium*, where mitotic divisions do not cease after emergence (*Devi et al.*, 1963), growth rate is, in contradistinction with *Drosophila*, positively correlated with adult longevity. This leads to the hypothesis that a faster growth rate, resulting probably in a shorter cellular life expectancy, must be associated in a certain number of stem cells with a higher potential number of cell divisions. The death of the individual will not coincide with the death of some particular cells but with the end of mitotic divisions in particular stem cells. Although some experimental attempts have been made, nothing is at present known about the *in vivo* limited or unlimited life-span of particular stem cells (*Reincke et al.,* 1975). However, one knows from *in vitro* studies that the number of generations through which fibroblast culture may be passed before the population senesces and dies out is reduced if the period of time between the subculturings is increased (*McHale et al.,* 1971). One may thus assume that a modification in mitotic rate, through a modification of an asymmetrical type of mitotic division (*Sheldrake,* 1974), may result in a modified cytoplasmic molecular composition or configuration. The possible importance of such cytoplasmic modification on the cellular fate was discussed above.

2. Programmed Cell Death

The existing links among growth rate, ageing and life-span in natural populations thus provide at least some indirect evidence in favour of a genetically programmed theory of ageing.

More direct evidence stems from the study of cellular death associated with morphogenesis. Cellular death occurs abundantly and predictably during embryogenesis. This is a normal component of most morphogenetic movements, such as foldings, detachment and the confluences of anlagen, and this occurs prominently during histogenesis. Moreover, this is the means whereby many embryonic and larval organs are eliminated during metamorphosis (reviews in *Glücksmann,* 1951; *Zwilling,* 1964).

The links among development, differentiation and ultimate death of the cell were emphasized as early as 1943 by the study of *Bodenstein* on the salivary glands of the larva of *D. virilis.* The larval salivary glands are strictly larval organs. They grow by increase in cell size and are completely histolysed during the early part of pupal life. More precisely, in response to metamorphic hormones, these glands are histolysed about 10 h after the formation of the puparium. These salivaries, however, possess the competence to respond by histolysis to the action of metamorphic hormones much earlier in life, i.e. immediately after the second moult. Indeed, when grafted to third instar larvae which are about to undergo metamorphosis, salivaries from second instar larvae are histolysed simultaneously with the salivaries of the host. This competence, however, is not present in the cells of the salivaries of larvae which have just completed the first moult. What competence is remains as yet an unsolved problem. That it is, at least partly, under genetical control is suggested by the study of the degenerative changes — mainly in the cochlea and the vestibular apparatus — which occur in mice affected by the classical waltzer-shaker syndrome. The developmental degeneration produced by the six or seven genes which produce the waltzer-shaker syndrome have been reviewed by *Grüneberg* (1956). It is clear that identical cellular degeneration may occur through the action of different genes, at the same or at different times of development, and at varying rates.

Another example pertains to the degeneration of the retinal photoreceptor cells in mice affected by retinal dystrophy. The disease is under control of a recessive gene. The retinal cells degenerate during days 11–18 of post-natal life (*Sorsby et al.*, 1954). Interestingly enough, retinal tissue from such mice explanted on the first post-natal day undergoes degeneration over the same period of time *in vitro* as it would have *in vivo* (*Hansson*, 1965). Clearly, genes may trigger a succession of events, the ultimate result of which is cellular death. This pattern of event has been referred to as a 'death clock' by *Saunders et al.* (1962). As rightly pointed by *Fallon and Saunders* (1968) it is, however, not clear whether mutations, such as the ones responsible for the waltzer-shaker syndrome or the retinal dystrophy, cause the differentiation of a 'death clock' where there is normally none, or possibly the converse, in such a way that the mutations allow a 'death clock' which is normally turned off to continue.

In this respect, evidence pertaining to cellular deaths which are a normal part of a regular developmental programme may yield more pertinent information. Experimental results obtained during the development of the chick embryo shows that both the competence to undergo cellular death and the developmental events which actually trigger its onset may be programmed. In the chick embryo, the occurrence of localized zones of intensive degeneration in the wing bud was shown to be correlated in space and time with the topographic distribution of prospective wing parts and with the morphogenetic movements which carve their definitive contours. Furthermore, grafting experiments have shown that the 'time of execution of the death sentence' in the tissues of the posterior necrotic zone of the wing bud is not modified by conditions resulting from heterochrony in the development of host and graft (*Saunders et al.*, 1962). Later on, an elegant, and unfortunately too rare, type of experiment, where *in vivo* and *in vitro* cell differentiation, ageing and death are compared, fully confirmed these results. Cells of the posterior necrotic zone of the chick embryo wing bud cultures *in vitro* in conditions that support normal growth and differentiation undergo necrosis on the same schedule as they do *in ovo*. This indicates that, as demonstrated for the posterior necrotic zone *in ovo*, these cells are 'programmed to die at an early stage of development'. How the programming occurs is as yet unknown, but the authors suspect that factors in the environment — intrinsic and extrinsic determinants, possibly similar to those that programme specific patterns of growth and biosynthesis for other cells — control the programming of the 'death clock'. Cellular death in this context appears to be fully integrated with other morphogenetic events and, in the words of the authors, 'the death of the posterior necrotic zone cells may be looked upon as an end-point for differentiation' (*Fallon and Saunders*, 1968; *Saunders and Fallon*, 1967).

In vivo observations of cellular, or rather tissular, deaths have also been made in cases where death does not probably make part of the normal fate of the cell line. We have noticed that *in vitro* cultures of normal, i.e. non-malignant or not transformed, diploid cells proliferate only for a limited number of cell generations. On the contrary, transformed cell lines may proliferate *ad infinitum*. Observations made on corresponding *in vivo* cell cultures give some ground to the idea that, at least to some extent, an intrinsic programme is responsible for the finite number of cell generations which a diploid normal cell culture may go through. Normal mice mammary gland tissue was serially transplanted in gland-free mammary fat pads of young female inbred mice. The growth of transplants was used as an index of ageing. The growth rate of normal gland declines with time and the oldest transplant line was lost after 2 years of serial passage. Interestingly enough, the growth of pre-neoplastic gland was not time-dependent and two such transplant lines were growing vigorously after more than 8 years in passage. The authors concluded that normal mammary gland has a limited ability to proliferate *in vivo*, even under favourable conditions, but that pre-neoplastic gland, like mammary tumours, has an apparently unlimited life-span when similarly propagated (*Daniel et al.*, 1968).

Williamson and Askonas (1972) confirmed these results. In mice, they propagated a single antibody-forming cell clone by serial transfer of limited numbers of spleen cells in inbred hosts. The continuing serial transfer experiment showed that the antibody-forming cell clone displayed a characteristic decline in proliferative capacity in response to repeated transplantation. It has a finite life-span. The authors further estimated that from the time of the first differentiation of the stem cell inducing it to be a progenitor of an antibody-forming cell clone, the overall proliferative potential is not more than 90 divisions. They have argued that this value was consistent with the life-span of cloned somatic cells *in vitro*.

Later on, *Daniel and Young* (1971), in a study of serial transfer of mice mammary gland tissues in gland-free mammary fat pads of female inbred mice, gathered evidence to the fact that the decline in growth rate of such transferred tissues is primarily related to the number of cell divisions undergone rather than to the passage of metabolic time. Their conclusions were primarily based on the comparison of the results of transplantations made at 3-month intervals with those at yearly intervals (fig. 14). In reality, a transplant of young mammary tissue placed in the center of a gland-free fat pad gives rise to a number of elongating ducts. 2 to 3 months are required for primary transplants to fill the fat pad. Afterwards, the resulting network of ducts remains mitotically quiescent.

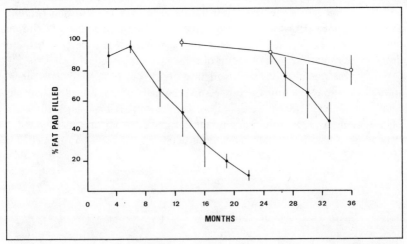

Fig. 14. Serial transplantation studies of mouse mammary gland. Two transplant lines were initiated from a single donor at time 0 and transplanted at intervals of 12 months (○) or 3 months (●). At 24 months, a second short-interval line was split from the 12-month series. 32 fat pads were transplanted at each generation. Vertical lines represent 95% confidence intervals. From *Daniel and Young* (1971).

The above data strongly suggest that cells have an intrinsic and predetermined capacity for division even under extremely favourable environmental conditions which favour growth. The capacity for division, the programme leading to death, may be modulated or drastically modified by mutation or by transformation, a phenomenon which, as we have seen (p. 39), is probably also of a genetic nature.

However, this is not the whole story. Extrinsic factors may also play a paramount role in the release of the death clock, acting as agents controlling the phenotypic expression of a genetically determined trait.

The experiments of *Fallon and Saunders* (1968) have shown that cells of the posterior necrotic zone of the chick embryo wing bud die *in vitro* on the same schedule as they do *in ovo*. Thus, this type of cell is apparently submitted to a programme of accelerated senescence. Under certain conditions, however, these cells may be diverted to a morphological fate involving continued life and eventual cytodifferentiation. Indeed, if competent posterior necrotic zone cells are grafted to the wing buds of a chick embryo, these cells not only show no sign of cellular degeneration but may eventually differentiate parallel to the development of the host embryo (*Saunders et al.,* 1962). In another experiment, competent posterior necrotic zone cells were placed transfilter to a large slice of central wing or leg mesoderm from a 3- to 4-day embryo. Again, the death of the cells fails to occur. The transfilter factor is as yet unidentified (*Fallon and Saunders*, 1968). However, the experiments show that products of the metabolism of a cell or of a group of cells may significantly interfere with the death programme of another cell or group of cells.

This was remarkably confirmed in a study of accelerated senescence provoked in low passage human embryonic lung cells of the W1-38 cell strain. The total cellular content of aged cells or of the cell wall of senescent cells was fractionated. A glycoprotein component extracted from the fractionated material causes almost immediate senescence when put on early passage cell cultures (*Milo*, 1973).

III. Genetics and Parental Age

The second problem which has to be faced is related to the potential importance of parental age on the faithful transmission of information from parent to offspring. A clear distinction must be made between the parental age related to characteristics of first generation progeny and the ability of such a progeny to transmit a distinctive pattern to successive generations (*Clark,* 1964; *Lints,* 1971). Therefore, we shall consider separately parental age effects and Lansing effects. We define parental age effects as the various outcome, transmissible or not, produced in the first generation offspring by one or a series of biological factors directly related to the age of the parents. Lansing effects are transmissible cumulative effects, whether reversible or not, due to the reproduction at a given time of the life cycle through successive parental generations; Lansing effects may reverse either spontaneously or when the reproduction pattern is modified (*Soliman and Lints,* 1976).

A. Parental Age Effects

The problem of parental age effects, for obvious reasons, has been thoroughly studied in man (reviews in *Cavalli-Sforza and Bodmer,* 1971; *Vogel and Rathenberg,* 1975; *Roberts and Bear,* 1977). The extreme differences between male spermatogenesis and female ovogenesis have in man some interesting implications. Really, if there is a constant rate of mutation in the gamete-producing cells, the frequency of mutant genes among male gametes should increase linearly with time. In females, as new egg cells are not formed after birth, there should be less opportunity for the accumulation of mutant genes.

Thus, in males two types of errors could be responsible for an increase of the mutation rate of gametes with increasing paternal age. Firstly, copying errors could occur during mitosis of the gamete-producing cells and accumulate with time; secondly, copying errors could occur during meiosis and, because of an eventual changing sensitivity of the spermatogonial cells, increase with advancing age. The situation in females is quite different, for they not only transfer a nucleus but also an important cytoplasmic material. Mutagenic agents of various kinds could of course accumulate mutations in resting ovocytes, but probably more important in relation with parental age effects is the fact that mature ovocytes contain a great amount of RNA and proteins produced by the maternal genome shortly before the maturation of the egg. No doubt that the production of such components, the role of which is paramount during embryological development, could be influenced by maternal age.

Directly related to the problem of differential gametogenesis is the very old and largely forgotten problem of rejuvenation. Recently, and with relevance to Hayflick's hypothesis of limited life-span of cells cultured *in vitro, Eaves* (1973) has restated the problem. He claims that the acceptance of the general validity of this hypothesis implies that the rejuvenation process takes place in the interval which starts at the onset of meiosis — where the germ cells have the age of their parents — and ends after fertilization — where the zygote is young.

1. Parental Age and Gametogenesis
a. In Man

In man, the conclusion which emerges from a review of the existing data related to parental age effects on mutation rates is not decisive. There are a few major genes whose mutation frequency is known to increase with paternal age, maternal age being of no influence. However, most of them show, either with paternal or maternal age, only minor variations, the significance of which is not always obvious. From a recent and exhaustive review of the existing data, *Vogel and Rathenberg* (1975) concluded, perhaps a bit uncautiously, that: 'The influence of paternal age on the mutation rate for a number of dominant conditions and one sex-linked recessive disease has been confirmed beyond any reasonable doubt ... However, the paternal age effect is not equally pronounced in all mutations. The mutations analyzed so far seem to fall into two categories. In one, the effect is strong and the slope of the curve becomes steeper from age group to age group. Examples of this group are achondroplasia, Apert's syndrome, myositis ossificans (fig. 15A), Marpan's syndrome and haemophilia A. The best example for the second group seems to be bilateral retinoblastoma (fig. 15B); however, there is some evidence that other conditions (tuberous sclerosis, neurofibromatosis, osteogenesis imperfecta) may behave in a similar manner.' However, as pointed out by *Roberts and Bear* (1977), it is still not clear whether there is a special sensitivity of male germ cells which increases with age or whether the age effect represents the accumulation of changes that occur through adult life. Moreover, it must be noted that the absence of any paternal age effect on observed mutation rates could simply be the reflection of a selective elimination of spermatogonial cells or of gametes containing a mutation.

On the other hand, chromosomal aberrations, resulting from dysfunction of meiosis — among which trisomy 21 has been thoroughly studied (fig. 16) — increase as a function of maternal age, paternal age having no influence at all. Hormonal imbalance has sometimes been considered as being the main cause of

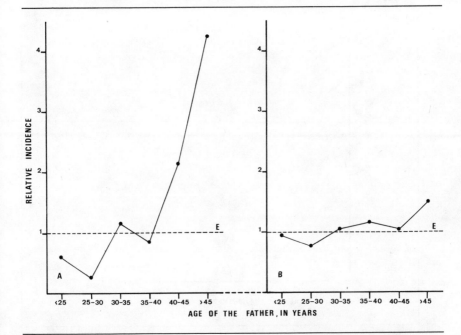

Fig. 15. Relative incidence of myositis ossificans (A) and bilateral retinoblastoma (B) as a function of the age of the father. Myositis ossificans progressiva is characterized by a distinctive pattern of ossification and of accompanying congenital deformation of hands and feet. It is due to a dominant mutation. Retinoblastoma, or glioma of the retina, which is caused by a dominant mutation, is a cancerous disease which originates in the retina of infants or very young children. The dashed line, marked E, indicates the expected value if no age dependence would exist. Compare the scale of the ordinate with the one of figure 16. Myositis ossificans: data from *Tünte et al.* (1967), redrawn from *Vogel and Rathenberg* (1975). Bilateral retinoblastoma: data from *Pellie et al.* (1973), redrawn from *Vogel and Rathenberg* (1975).

these errors of meiosis. One may wonder, however, how far the ageing of the ovocytes I, all formed during the early stages of embryogenesis, may bring some modifications in the cytoplasmic molecular composition or configuration, the result of which is an irregular meiosis!

b. Discontinuous Variation

The very same reason could be, and has been, invoked to explain some almost forgotten experimental results of *Bridges* (1927, 1929). In *D. melanogaster, Bridges* studied the percentage of recombination for seven loci of chromosome III in successive 2-day broods during the entire life of a certain number of females. This study showed that the percentages of recombination varied in a

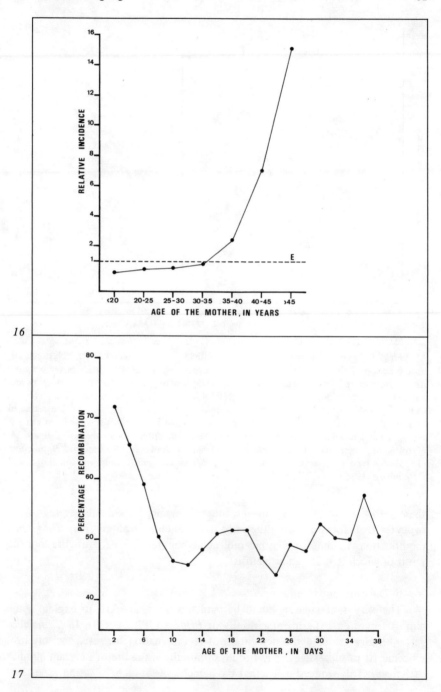

16

17

Table XV. Effect of maternal age on the percentage of recombination in mice

Age, months	Number of mice observed	Recombinants	
		number	%
2	115	37	32.2
3	84	26	30.9
4	106	26	24.5
5	98	28	28.6
6	108	37	34.3
7	73	17	23.3
8	92	22	23.9
9–10	80	18	22.5
>10	49	10	20.4

Modified from *Bodmer* (1961).

The linear regression of recombination fraction with increasing maternal age is significant at the 0.05 level. Female coupling and repulsion heterozygotes, $\frac{pa\ fi}{+\ +}$ and $\frac{pa\ +}{+\ fi}$, were back-crossed to double recessive males. Palled (pa) and fidget (fi) are two recessive genes situated in the linkage group V.

regular and cyclic way – as shown by the sum of the separate percentages (fig. 17). Later on, notably in the present respect, an almost unknown paper of *Bergner* (1928) provided evidence that modifications in the length of the pre-imaginal period of life obtained by various manipulations of the environment in turn modified the imaginal cycle of variation in crossover frequency. The results of *Bridges* have been recently confirmed by *Valentin* (1973) in a study of selection for altered recombination frequency in *D. melanogaster*. Variations in the amount of recombination with maternal age have also been observed in mice (table XV) (*Fisher*, 1949; *Bodmer*, 1961). It is not impossible that the meiotic

Fig. 16. Relative incidence of Down's syndrome in man as a function of the age of the mother. Down's syndrome, formerly called mongolism, is due to the trisomy of chromosome 21. The dashed line, marked E, indicates the expected value if no age dependence would exist. Data from *Penrose and Smith* (1966), recalculated from figure 3.6 in *Cavalli-Sforza and Bodmer* (1971).

Fig. 17. Sum of six separate percentages of recombination as a function of the age of the mother for seven loci of chromosome III of *D. melanogaster*. The separate percentages of recombination are calculated from the observation of the offspring of eight isolated females of the genotype:

$$\frac{ru + D + p^b + c^s}{+\ h + st + ss +},$$

crossed with sextuple recessive males. A total of 15,544 offspring was observed. Redrawn from *Bridges* (1929).

Table XVI. Effects of the age of the mother on the characteristics of the guinea pig

Age of mother months	Amount of white spotting, % white		Occurrence of polydactyly, %
	female	male	
3–6	60.5	56.3	52.7 ± 1.8
6–9	67.6	59.5	40.0 ± 1.7
9–12	66.5	60.6	29.2 ± 1.7
12–15	70.6	61.3	26.7 ± 1.7
15–21	69.6	63.2	18.5 ± 1.4
21–46	73.3	66.9	14.2 ± 1.4

Modified from *Wright* (1926).
In highly inbred lines of guinea pigs, the amount of white spotting increases with the age of the mother. On the contrary, the occurrence of polydactyly decreases sharply as a function of mother's age.

Table XVII. Influence of maternal age on the incidence – expressed in percent – of various skeletal anomalies in the mouse

Age of the mother, days	Cranial dystopia	Dystopia sacrum	Caudal dystopia	Absence of lower third molar
<130	6.3	34.7	[10.9	6.3
130–160	5.0	22.9	[	3.2
160–190	4.5	11.3	[	[
190–220	1.1	19.4	2.6	
220–250	0.0	13.2		0.0
>250	0.0	8.1	[	[

Modified from *Searle* (1954).

irregularities which increase with maternal age and the variations in crossover frequency which decrease with maternal age are provoked by a common factor. Early work with *Drosophila* showed a clear relationship between non-disjunction and recombination (*Mather,* 1938). An increase of non-disjunction is generally associated with a decrease in crossover frequency, and the two have a common origin in the restriction of pairing at meiosis. The origin of such restriction in pairing still remains obscure.

Some observations of *Wright* (1926) indicate that purely environmental influences, or rather non-genetic factors, linked to maternal age, may have a profound effect on the expression of a gene or of a group of genes. *Wright* studied the influence of maternal age on the amount of white spotting and the occurrence of polydactyly in highly inbred lines of guinea pigs. Most, if not all, of the observed variations in such strains are thus due to non-genetic factors. The piebald pattern of coloured spots on a white ground depends on an incompletely recessive gene. The polydactyly probably depends on four pairs of alleles but could also depend on one major gene and an unknown number of polygenes (*Wright,* 1960). The amount of white spotting increases with the age of the female and most of the variation is due to non-genetic factors which are different even in litter mates. The percentage of polydactyly decreases considerably with maternal age, and more than half of the non-genetic variation is due to factors common to litter mates, in contrast with the situation in the case of the piebald pattern (table XVI). Anyhow, the non-genetic environmental influence on gene expression, due to maternal age, is here perfectly evident.

The same type of evidence has been obtained by *Searle* (1954) in a study of the influence of maternal age on the development of the skeleton of the mouse. *Searle* studied only highly inbred lines, where variations are still extensive, which shows the paramount importance of non-genetic factors on the expression of a given set of genes. He examined the incidence of 21 anomalies in two strains. Most of the total variance, over 80% in three quarters of the characters, is due to intangible non-genetic factors acting independently on individuals or sides of individuals. But significant trends with maternal age occur in seven out of the 21 anomalies, accounting on the average for about 10% of the total variance with respect to these seven (table XVII).

c. Continuous Variation

It will be clear to all biologists that the sort of variation just discussed, i.e. linked to the action of a single or a small number of so-called major genes or, eventually, to gross chromosomal rearrangements, embraces only a small part of the variation which occurs in nature. The differences which characterize natural populations and which make that individuals among a species so widely differ from each other are rarely matters of nature, but are nearly all matters of degree. Variations of this sort, i.e. continuous variation, depend both on genetic and non-genetic causes. The genetic part of the determination of such traits depends on the simultaneous segregation of many genes, the so-called minor genes or polygenes, while the non-genetic part depends on the action of a set of environmental causes. Therefore, it is not useless to examine to what an extent parental age influences the phenotypic expression of quantitative traits of the offspring.

There is a good number of published evidence about subtle differences in growth, development, longevity and various other quantitative traits between the offspring of young and old parents (reviews in *Strong,* 1954; *Parsons,* 1964; partial reviews in *Lints and Hoste,* 1974, 1977). Such evidence, however, is difficult to interpret. This results from the fact that most of the experimentalists observed the progeny of ageing parents only at two or three moments, more or

Table XVIII. Means ± standard error of thoracic size (in mm), duration of development (in days) and three indices of the fecundity for first generation offspring of *D. melanogaster* females reproduced when young and old. Note that the offspring of older parents have a shorter duration of development, a smaller size and a much higher fecundity than offspring of younger parents. The very same flies have been used for reproduction at young (4 days after emergence, at 25 °C) and old age (26 days). The parental age effect is tested by means of analysis of variance

Item	Parental age at reproduction		Parental age effects	
	young	old	variance ratio	signif-icance
Thoracic size	1.008 ± 0.006	1.036 ± 0.008	F^1_{76}	23.9	<0.001
Duration of development	9.48 ± 0.07	8.74 ± 0.07	$F^1_{1,192}$	167	<0.001
Total fecundity	1,576 ± 205	2,522 ± 65	F^1_8	19.2	<0.001
Mean daily egg production	36.9 ± 2.9	51.1 ± 4.3	F^1_8	7.6	<0.05
Maximal daily egg production	89.0 ± 4.3	113.6 ± 6.0	F^1_8	10.6	<0.05

Modified from *Lints and Hoste* (1974, 1977) and *Hoste* (1975).

less randomly chosen, of the parental life-time. This follows from the *a priori* belief, which closely follows the interpretation of *Lansing* (1954) (see p. 79 devoted to the Lansing effects), that parental age effects are a linear function of parental age, i.e. that they are absent when the parents are young and that they appear and increase as the parents grow older. However, it is clear, in a certain number of cases, and at least in insects, that when a given trait is measured in all successive daily progenies of ageing pairs, the trait appears to vary in a cyclic rather than in a linear way. Such are, for instance in *D. melanogaster,* the variations of the size of the egg (*David,* 1959, 1962; *Parsons,* 1962; *Delcour,* 1969), of the number of abdominal bristles (*Wattiaux and Heuts,* 1963), of the sternopleural chaeta number asymmetry (*Parsons,* 1962), of wing size (*Delcour and Heuts,* 1968), of development time (*Delcour,* 1969), of the sum of the percentages of recombination for seven loci of chromosome III (*Bridges,* 1927), of the relative percentages of different genotypes obtained from dihybrid backcrosses (*Heuts,* 1956), of the RNA and DNA content of virgin eggs (*Tsien and Wattiaux,* 1971).

Thus, it may be accepted without any doubt that the offspring of young and old parents differ for a variety of quantitative characters. These variations may be linear as a function of parental age, but are probably cyclic. However, in spite of the great number of published observations, the evidence is not always easy to interpret. Indeed, the first hypothesis which comes to mind to explain such results is that offspring from old parents are offspring from a selected long-living, and thus possibly genetically different, component of the base population. Such a hypothesis can in general hardly be rejected on the basis of the published evidence. Indeed, some authors use different groups of adults to yield offspring from young and old parents. Some others do not say anything about the relationship between the young and old parents. A few experiments are, however, not subject to such criticism. They indeed show that parental age effects are due to ageing. Such are the experiments where the young and the old parents are identical (table XVIII) (*Lints and Hoste,* 1974, 1977; *Hoste,* 1975) and experiments where the successive daily offspring of ageing *single* pairs are observed. The number of abdominal bristles (*Wattiaux and Heuts,* 1963), the wing size (*Delcour and Heuts,* 1968) and the cell size and cell number of the wing (*Delcour,* 1969) of *D. melanogaster* were observed in this way in the successive progenies of single pairs of flies. All these traits were shown to vary in a cyclic rather than in a linear way as a function of parental age.

d. Relative Parental Age

In the case of age-dependent cyclic variations in wing size, the curves of variations of single pairs are found to be synchronous when the data are plotted as a function of relative maternal age (fig. 18) (*Delcour and Heuts,* 1968). This is consistent with the hypothesis that the successive events of the life cycle are proportionately accelerated or decelerated with the length of maternal life.

The biological meaning of the notion of relative age is clearly thrown into relief by the recalculation of some data pertaining to the influence of parental age at reproduction on the progeny life-span in *Paramecium aurelia. P. aurelia,* a ciliated protozoan which possesses two micronuclei and one macronucleus, has a well-defined life cycle where the following phases can be easily identified: sexual immaturity, maturity, senescence and death. *P. aurelia* reproduces by fission, which is a mitotic process, or by a meiotic process, either autogamy or conjugation. During the meiotic process of reproduction, which initiates a new life cycle, the micronuclei undergo meiosis, one haploid gamete reproduces itself, there is a mutual exchange of gametes during conjugation or a fusion of genetically identical gametes in autogamy and the zygote nucleus develops to new macro- and micronuclei for the progeny clones. In short, clones which undergo successive mitotic divisions age and die, but when these clones initiate progeny clones by undergoing autogamy or conjugation they assure, so to say, the 'immortality' of the species. During the maturity period of a clone, it is easy to force one of the fission products of a cell to undergo autogamy and thus to initiate a new progeny clone, while the other fission product proceeds to divide mitotically. (For full details concerning the biology of *P. aurelia,* see *Sonneborn,* 1974.)

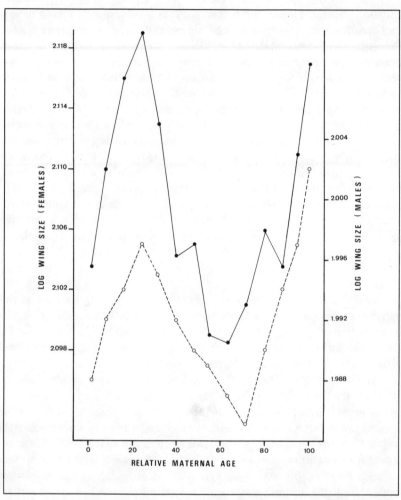

Fig. 18. Variations of the wing size (in log values) in female (•) and male (○) *D. melanogaster* as a function of maternal age. The wing size values of the successive daily progenies of eleven single ageing pairs of Oregon × Swedish B *D. melanogaster* are synchronized on the basis of the hypothesis of an acceleration or deceleration of the successive events of maternal life proportional to the length of that life. Redrawn with permission from *Delcour and Heuts* (1968).

Smith-Sonneborn et al. (1974) made use of these various possibilities to study the influence of parental age, i.e. the number of fissions since the origin of the clone at autogamy, on the progeny life-span, i.e. the number of fissions from origin to the death of the clone. More precisely, they studied the progeny life-span, firstly, in relation with the parental fission age at the origin, by autogamy, of the progeny clone and, secondly, in relation with the parental life-span, i.e. the total number of fissions that the parental strain undergoes before dying. They found that 'progeny life-span decreased with increasing parental age and that parental life-span was a significant variable in the determination of progeny life-span'.

We have calculated (*Stoll,* 1977; *Lints and Stoll,* in preparation) the regression between the progeny life-span and the parental age at reproduction and found it significant, although only 27% of the variance is explained by the regression (fig. 19A). However, when the same data pertaining to the progeny life-span are plotted as a function of the relative parental age (i.e. the number of parental fissions at the origin of the progeny clone with regard to the number of parental fissions at the death of the parental clone), 67% of the variance is explained by the regression. Finally, when the data concerning the parental clones which do not live for more than 100 fissions – an extremely short life-span which could be due to the effect of a few detrimental genes – are excluded, the regression explains as much as 85% of the variance (fig. 19B).

From this set of data it may be safely deduced that, for a given species, the succession of events which characterize a life cycle – the programme! – may be unreeled at different speeds. This implies that, on the average, for a given set of individuals of that species, the distances between the events of their respective life cycles are lengthened or shortened proportionally to their respective life-spans (p. 85).

e. Heritability

For a variety of quantitative traits, the phenotypic expression of the offspring thus varies as a function of parental age. That these variations are, most probably and at least partly, due to a variation in the information content of the gametes of ageing parents is strongly suggested by a series of recent studies on the variations of heritability in relation to parental age. Heritability estimates the degree of resemblance between relatives. For a particular trait, it expresses the proportion of the total phenotypic variance that is genetic. (Strictly speaking: the proportion that is additive genetic variance.) Heritability is commonly expressed in percentage and thus decreases with an increasing environmental component of variance.

In *D. melanogaster,* the heritability of sternopleural chaeta number is influenced by the age of the parents such that estimates based upon parents of 14 days and more are significantly greater than those from 3-day-old parents. The age effect on heritability is more marked with age of the mother, but there is also a male effect (*Beardmore et al.,* 1975; *Lints and Beardmore,* 1975). In the guppy-fish, *Poecilia reticulata,* the same type of evidence has been obtained for the number of caudal fin-rays (*Beardmore and Shami,* 1976). Furthermore, a

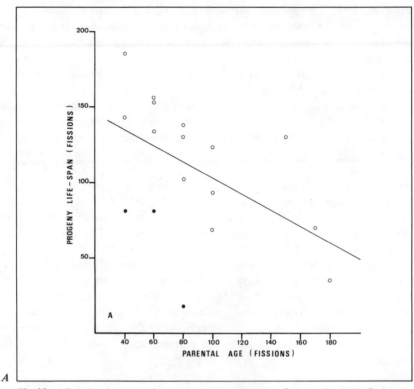

A

Fig. 19. A Relation between the parental age — number of parental mitotic fissions at the origin, by autogamy, of the offspring clone — and the progeny life-span — mean number, for five to eight replicates, of mitotic fissions at the death of the clone — in *P. aurelia*. The regression is of the form y = 156.3 − 0.54x, with a correlation coefficient r = − 0.512 (n = 18; p <0.05). The regression thus explains 27% of the offspring variance. *B* The regression between progeny life-span and the relative parental age — in percent, transformed into degrees — is of the form y = 237.8 − 2.58x with a correlation coefficient r = − 0.818 (n = 18; p <0.001). When the three points (●) relating to the parental life-span of 100 fissions — a particularly low number of fissions! due to the influence of a few deleterious genes? — are excluded, the regression is of the form y = 241.0 − 2.46x, and the correlation coefficient r = −0.923 (n = 15; p <0.001) which means that 85% of the offspring variance is explained by the regression. Calculated and drawn with permission from tables I and II in *Smith-Sonneborn et al.* (1974).

re-analysis of the *D. melanogaster* data has shown that the age-dependent effects on heritability are found mainly in parents with central phenotypes for the trait investigated, and which are probably more heterozygous, and not for those with extreme phenotypes, which are probably more homozygous (*Shami,* 1977).

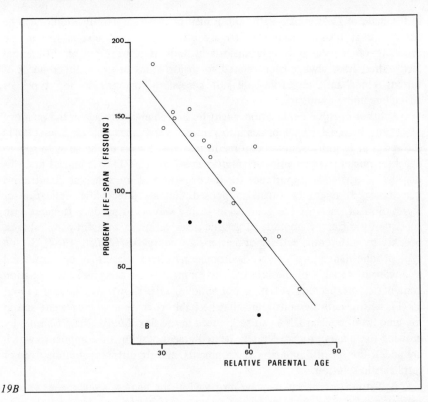

19B

These heritability studies bear direct relation with the stochastic theories of ageing. Indeed, in relation with the error-catastrophe theory of ageing, and with other related theories, it could be argued that if heritability were to change with parental age it would be more likely to decrease than to increase. In actuality, if there was an accumulation of mutational errors in meiotic cells, the resemblance between parents and offspring for a phenotypic character with a value fixed at a point in early life — as bristle number in *Drosophila* or finger ridges in man — should diminish with age. But this is not so.

Various hypotheses may be put forward to explain the parental age-dependent increase in heritability: variations of the amount of recombination, of meiotic drive or affinity, of the quantity of genetic material or of gene-controlling elements which pass into gametes.

The observed increase in heritability with parental age could be attributed to a decrease in the amount of recombination during parental gametogenesis. However, the existence of a paternal effect suggests that reduced recombination, even if it applies, cannot be the whole of the story, as there is no recombination in the male of *Drosophila*. Variation in meiotic drive or affinity should also be considered as possible causes of an age effect. However, inequalities in the products of female and male meiosis as well as some cases of differential fertilization have always been related to major genes or gross disturbances of various kinds and, therefore, are not necessarily relevant to the types of characters under discussion.

Another possible explanation might lie in a change with age in the quantity of genetic material which passes into gametes. *Darlington and La Cour* (1941) showed that in mitosis, heterochromatin may not always divide so as to pass to daughter nuclei in equal amounts. *Mather and Jinks* (1971) have argued that this may be of particular importance for the evolution of the genes of quantitative inheritance. It might be further supposed that age affects the replication or segregation of parts of the genome in such a way as to produce gametes with consistently different amounts of genetic information at different parental ages, possibly by differential activity of master-slave complexes (*Callan,* 1967). Such a type of inheritance involving an environmental effect — age may be considered as a relevant variable of the internal environment — on the genetic information content is unexpected; yet it is not unique, as is shown by *Durrant* (1962, 1971), who clearly demonstrated that heritable changes in plant weight and in the amount of nuclear DNA can be induced in the flax, *Linum usitatissimum,* by growing the plants in a moderately heated greenhouse in soil compost to which are added the specific inducing environments, namely different combinations of fertilizers in solution.

A further hypothesis may be proposed in the light of some recent experimental results. The analysis of the variation of heritability as a function of parental age has been done, both in *P. reticulata* and in *D. melanogaster,* on ageing *populations.* This means essentially that the heritability variation observed in such populations may be due to two factors acting either in an additive or in an opposite way. The first factor would depend on the age of the *individuals* tested; the second on the changing genetic structure of the ageing *population.* The genetic structure of a population, as defined by a system of gene and genotype frequencies, may influence the estimate of heritability. As we have seen, heritability expresses the proportion of the total phenotypic variance that is genetic; thus, it decreases with an increasing environmental component of variance or with a decreasing genetic component of variance. It may thus be safely assumed that heritability will increase in an ageing population where the amount of heterozygotes increases at the expense of homozygotes.

For a certain time, it was suspected (*Lerner,* 1954) that the more heterozygous the individuals the longer they may eventually survive. In other words, in a given population the first deaths could occur among the more homozygous individuals. For instance — but there are numerous other examples of the same nature — *Dobzhansky and Wallace* (1953) compared the survival

Table XIX. Analysis of total finger ridge count (TFRC) in a twin study in man. Influence of maternal age at conception on the within-pair TFRC differences in monozygotic (MZ) and dizygotic (DZ) twins, on the within-pair TFRC correlation coefficients and on the estimates of heritability. Heritability is calculated from the equation $h^2 = r_{MZ} - r_{DZ}/1 - C$ *(Jensen,* 1967). 558 twins, i.e. 279 pairs of all sex and zygosity combinations have been analyzed

Maternal age	Within-pair TFRC differences		Within-pair TFRC correlation coefficients		Heritability
	MZ	DZ	MZ	DZ	
<28 years	11.64	31.71	0.925	0.568	0.714
28–33	8.17	32.96	0.980	0.544	0.871
>33 years	6.62	34.33	0.986	0.507	0.957

Modified from *Lints et al.* (1976).

rates in replicate cultures of various, artificially created, homozygotes and heterozygotes for certain chromosomes from populations of *D. pseudoobscura, D. persimilis, D. prosaltans* and *D. melanogaster.* The survival rates were found to be higher in heterozygotes than in homozygotes in all four species. Likewise, the mean viability of homozygotes was lower than that of heterozygotes.

It is probable that this conclusion may be extended reasonably to natural populations. Indeed, in *P. reticulata, Shami* (1977) has shown that ageing populations are characterized by a significant reduction in the phenotypic variance of the two metric characters that he analyzed, i.e. number of caudal fin rays and lateral line scale number. The reduction in phenotypic variance is accompanied by an increase of heterozygotes at four polymorphic enzyme loci as shown by electrophoretic assay.

We therefore suggest that the heritability increase observed in ageing populations may be due to a changing ratio of heterozygotes versus homozygotes. This does not mean that the other hypotheses discussed above are to be rejected. They may explain, totally or partly, the age effect on heritability either on ageing populations or on ageing individuals.

Finally, the age effect on heritability may also be considered in terms of gene control. If it is so, it may mean two things. Firstly, the information related to genetic control systems varies with the age of the parents in such a way that the older the parents, the better the phenotypic expression of a given set of polygenes in the offspring, i.e. this expression is less influenced by non-genetic factors. Secondly, it could also be assumed that the additivity of action of a given set of polygenes, which determines a quantitative trait, is increased when transmitted by older parents.

In man, through a twin study, we have investigated the variations of heritability of the total finger ridge count (TFRC), a quantitative trait easy to measure and which is known to be determined largely by genetic factors (*Holt*, 1968). Both the average within-pair TFRC difference and the heritability of the trait have been analyzed. The average difference between the co-twins' TFRC appears to undergo a regular and remarkable decrease in monozygotic twin pairs, who are genetically identical, with increasing maternal age at conception, whereas an opposite trend is found for dizygotes, who are genetically different (table XIX). In the case of the paternal age, the trend is not equally clear, although this is again inverse for monozygotic and dizygotic twins. The analysis of the within-pair correlation coefficients confirms the observed trends: the correlations between monozygotic twin partners increase with maternal age at conception, whereas those between dizygotic twin partners decrease (table XIX). Finally, the analysis of heritability, carried out with different methods, clearly confirms these results: it increases with maternal age (table XIX) (*Lints et al.*, 1976; *Lints and Parisi*, 1977).

The study of the heritability of TFRC in man may, we feel, give some ground to the hypothesis which considers the age effect on heritability in terms of gene control. Indeed, it is not only the heritability which varies with age; the phenotypic expression of the trait varies also with parental age. More precisely, monozygotic twins, which are genetically identical, resemble each other more and more as parental age increases. In contrast, dizygotic twins, which are genetically different, i.e. their resemblance is not more than that of normal sibs, differ phenotypically more and more from each other as parental age increases. We believe that this strongly suggests that a given set of genes, responsible for a precise quantitative trait, is better expressed and its expression is less modified by environmental influences in proportion to the increase in parental age. A last point should be stressed: the data pertaining to an age effect on heritability are still insufficient to ascertain definitively that the age effect is or not linear as a function of parental age.

f. Conclusions

Three conclusions emerge from the examination of data relating to parental age effects on first generation progeny. Firstly, except for traits which are related directly to genetic 'accidents' — namely mutations, chromosomal non-disjunction, and so on — which *may* vary in a linear way in relation to maternal and/or paternal age, most quantitative traits probably vary in a non-linear way, showing one or more peaks during the life cycle of the parents. The optimal age for reproduction is not the earliest age (*Parsons*, 1964; *Lints*, 1971). Secondly, gametes produced by parents of different ages are different from one another in a systematic rather than a random way, for which, despite a recent speculation about its possible mechanism, no clear explanation is yet available (*Sheldrake*,

1974). However, the systematic and regularly non-linear variations of the gametes as a function of parental age clearly plead against the hypothesis which says that parental age effects are due to the accumulation of changes which occur through a life cycle and which attributes such changes to copying errors with a constant probability per DNA replication. Thirdly, the successive events of a life cycle may be proportionately accelerated or decelerated as a function of the length of life.

2. Rejuvenation

If Hayflick's hypothesis regarding the limited life-span of cell cultures *in vitro* has to be taken for granted, and if it applies as well to the life-span of cell strains *in vivo* — we have seen that there are some serious doubts about the general validity of both these points — germ cells, up to meiosis, have the age of their bearers. Of course, immediately after meiosis and fertilization, the newly formed zygote is young. This implies, as stated by *Eaves* (1973), that a rejuvenation process has taken place somewhere between the onset of meiosis and the beginning of development.

Rejuvenation, in theory, may apply to the cytoplasm, the nucleus or to both cytoplasm and nucleus. The evidence available may be interpreted in favour of a narrow interdependence between cytoplasmic and nuclear ageing. It does not allow to conclude that only one of the two elements, cytoplasm or nucleus, would be rejuvenated nor to decide whether the cytoplasm or the nucleus would actually be rejuvenated.

However, a choice has been made, at least implicitly, by a number of theoreticians of ageing. To claim that ageing is exclusively due to the expression of specific genetic events such as ageing genes or to the exhaustion of genetic information amounts to saying that rejuvenation must be nuclear. On the contrary, to affirm that the gradual accumulation and the subsequent catastrophic concentration of random errors in proteins responsible for transcription or translation implies that the cytoplasm controls senescence and should therefore be rejuvenated at the beginning of a new life cycle.

a. Cytoplasmic Rejuvenation

Cytoplasmic senescence factors and rejuvenation of the cytoplasm are apparent in some of the experiments reported by *Jinks* (1954, 1956) and *Mather and Jinks* (1958). For example: *Aspergillus glaucus* is a filamentous fungus which can be propagated either from the tips of the hyphae, or from conidia which are asexual spores, or from ascospores which are sexually produced. Now, if propagation is carried out for several generations by asexual conidia, the production of ascospores gradually decreases up to a point where the fungus completely loses its capacity for sexual reproduction. The same occurs when the reproduction is dependent upon hyphal tips and the capacity for reproduction

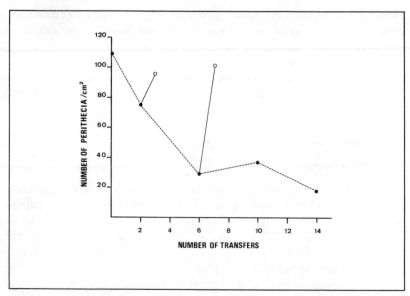

Fig. 20. The effects of propagation by conidia and by ascospores on the production of perithecia in *A. glaucus.* The continued propagation by conidia (-----) results in a decline of perithecial production. This decrease is progressive. It is not impredictable as it would be in case of alterations produced by nuclear gene mutations. On the contrary, it appears as due to cytoplasmic alterations, characteristic of a normal process of differentiation and development. In *A. glaucus* the production of perithecia is immediately restored to its original level by a single propagation through an ascospore (———). In *A. nidulans (Jinks,* 1954) the improvement in perithecial formation is gradual and proceeds during several generations of transfers by ascospores. Redrawn with permission from *Mather and Jinks* (1958).

of conidia is also lost. But until the sexual capacity of producing ascospores is completely lost, the fungus may be restored to complete sexuality through a single sexual propagation through an ascospore (fig. 20). Similar changes have been observed in *Neurospora (Sheng,* 1951).

Thus, when the reproduction is asexual, either by conidia or hyphal tips, it appears that only capacities essential to the operative reproductive cycle are retained, the cytoplasm changing so as to lose the ability for sustaining types of development no longer significant to the organism. With continued sexual propagation, the production of conidia is of no more importance than is that of ascospores with conidial propagation, yet conidia are never lost as a result of sexual propagation. In contrast to the asexual, the sexual cycle maintains in the cytoplasm the full range of developmental capacities even when they are no longer of significance. Furthermore, the plant can be restored to complete sexuality by a single propagation through an ascospore coming after a long period of asexual reproduction. In the words of *Mather and Jinks* (1958): 'Evidently the process of sexual reproduction involves a positive readjustment of the cytoplasm, a "spring-cleaning" or "retailoring" so that despite the alterations the standard basic cytoplasmic pattern is once again restored. There has been a cytoplasmic progression during the time of asexual propagation but it is brought full circle during the process of sexual reproduction.'

b. Nuclear Rejuvenation

The fact that the cytoplasm plays a paramount role not only in the process of differentiation and development but also, and in a similar manner, in the process of ageing is further ascertained by a rare study of the cytoplasmic induction of changes in the ultrastructure of the nucleus and the perinuclear cytoplasm of *Acetabularia mediterranea* (*Berger and Schweiger*, 1975). *A. mediterranea* is a giant single-celled alga. The zygote is derived from the fusion of two isogametes. It germinates to form a stalk. At its apical end, it forms a persistent cap, while at the posterior end a rhizoid is formed which contains the single nucleus. The total length of the cell may be 3—5 cm and this is reached within 3 months. An additional month is needed for the formation of a full-grown cap. Cells of *Acetabularia* thus display conspicuous morphological changes during their life cycle. But besides the macroscopic changes, a number of differences in the fine structure of the cell nucleus can be observed as well. These changes are most pronounced in the nucleolus and the perinuclear cytoplasm. (For full details concerning macroscopic and ultrastructural changes related to ageing in *A. mediterranea,* see *Haemmerling,* 1963; *Berger and Schweiger,* 1973; *Franke et al.,* 1974.)

Berger and Schweiger implanted nuclei from old cells into the cytoplasm of young cells, and vice versa. An old cell is one which has formed a cap of maximum diameter, while a young cell is one of about 1 cm. When a nucleus of an old cell is implanted into the cytoplasm of a young cell, that nucleus is rejuvenated; it assumes the typical morphology of a young nucleus within less than 10 days. On the contrary, the cytoplasm of an old cell is able to induce the reverse change in the implanted nucleus from a young cell. The cytoplasmic induction of nuclear ageing proceeds more rapidly than nuclear rejuvenation. In a certain number of cases, particularly important in young stalks into which old nuclei had been implanted (and this could be important), no nuclei were found when they were searched after a certain time of implantation.

These findings clearly show that the cytoplasmic state has an influence on the cell nucleus. Furthermore, the fact that an unusually high number of old nuclei are lost after implantation could mean either that after a certain stage of development a nucleus cannot be switched back to a young state, or that, on the model of the incompatibility which exists between cytoplasm and nucleus of some related species, there exists in a given species an incompatibility between an old nucleus and a young cytoplasm.

c. Nucleo-Cytoplasmic Interactions

The nucleo-cytoplasmic interactions which affect gene expression have been mostly investigated from the point of view of the nuclear influence on the cytoplasm. The reverse situation has attracted less attention. The necessity of rejuvenation or retailoring of the cytoplasm and the cytoplasmic induction of the rejuvenation or ageing of the nucleus (how both processes are mediated remains unknown) imply that the cytoplasm contains information-bearing constituents which have an influence on development, differentiation, ageing and on such essential processes as absence or presence of fertilization. Of course, the cytoplasm will not age without information sent by the nucleus. But once that information has been sent and received, it probably generates or controls ageing changes both in the cytoplasm and the nucleus.

Such an idea is of course not novel. It was indeed advocated – in a slightly different context – by *Gurdon*. He believes that the cytoplasmic control of nuclear activity during animal development is due to cytoplasmic components with a regulatory role. These components become associated with the chromosomes at a stage of mitosis where the nuclear membrane is absent and the chromosomes are necessarily exposed to the cytoplasm. This would constitute a reprogramming of chromosomal genes and would account for a subsequent change of nuclear function in mitosis. The argument may reasonably be extended to the chromosomes-cytoplasm association during mitosis. According to this suggestion, the components which regulate nuclear function could be synthesized in the cytoplasm prior to the mitosis or the meiosis at which they would become effective (*Gurdon and Woodland,* 1968), i.e. at different periods of the parental life cycle.

Yet, it is well known that in amphibians, echinoderms, nematodes, molluscs and insects, among others (review in *Brown and Dawid,* 1969) where the embryo plus abundant nutrient material constitutes a separate developing unit, RNA and protein products of maternal gene action are synthesized, stored and released at specific times and places. Mature oocytes, after fertilization, are transcriptionally inactive, maternal mRNA and ribosomes being present, and translation starts from stored mRNA and ribosome complexes. Therefore, most, if not all, embryos depend for their early development, and in some cases for the development of much later stages, on material stored in the oocyte cytoplasm (*Snow,* 1976). Variations in the composition of the oocyte cytoplasm may therefore affect to a greater or lesser extent the development and later differentiation of the embryo.

One may thus venture to speculate that the genetic material of developing individuals derived from parents of different ages is differentially activated either through products of translation or through the release of stored gene products or/and, as suggested by *Wolpert*'s (1969) theory of positional information, through the action of localized morphogenetic substances.

B. Lansing Effects

Most of the observations about parental age effects have been made only during one or, exceptionally, two generations and are therefore in the present respect of no help. Are these parental age effects transmissible, cumulative and irreversible? Are they transmissible, cumulative, reversible either naturally or through a modification of the age at reproduction?

If they are transmissible, cumulative and irreversible they should be due to some permanent modification in the genetic information system or in the lecture system. It may well then be argued that the variations in growth, development and longevity observed in relation to parental age are due to permanent changes in information-bearing or lecture system. Ageing and death could then also be related to such permanent changes: the mutation or derived theories of ageing would then at least be strengthened.

Now if, on the contrary, these effects are transmissible, cumulative and reversible, it implies that the observed variations are due to some non-permanent modifications in information-bearing, control or lecture systems. In other words, the sequence of events, the sum of which constitutes development, differentiation and ageing are modified, accelerated or decelerated because some constituents of the gametes or zygotes are modified as a function of parental age. These constituents, through some form of interaction or of differential activation of the genetic material or some type of information-bearing material, could accelerate or decelerate development and ageing. This in turn would suggest that ageing and death are not necessarily due to stochastic modifications of the genetic information or of the lecture system, in the strict sense of the word, but could be due to sequential and coordinated events, linked to development, the course of which is determined by the original constitution, in the broadest sense of the word, of the zygote. Indeed, the remarkable work of the embryologists of the beginning of the century has amply demonstrated that modifications of the first sequential events or embryogenesis have a profound influence on the subsequent stages of development (for reviews, see *Davidson*, 1968; *Løvtrup*, 1974).

1. The Cumulative Parental Age Effects

a. Lansing's Experiments in *Philodina citrina*

The first and most famous experiments involving the transmission of parental age effects are those of *Lansing* (1947, 1948, 1956). He was inspired by

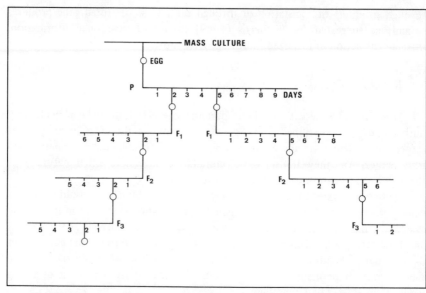

Fig. 21. Orthoclone method, showing the procedure developed by *Lansing* for selecting successive generations of a parthenogenetic rotifer, *P. citrina* or *E. triquetia,* with constant parental age in each generation. The two particular cases illustrated yield respectively a 2-day and a 5-day orthoclone. Redrawn with permission from *Lansing* (1947).

the pioneer work of *Jennings and Lynch* (1928). He used the parthenogenetic rotifers, *P. citrina* and *Euchlanis triquetra.* He clearly demonstrated a cumulative maternal age effect on the life-span and overall fitness of the offspring. However, Lansing effects are wrongly considered to be synonymous with detrimental cumulative parental age effects: the older the age of the orthoclone – an orthoclone is a series of successive generations with a uniform parental age (fig. 21) – the greater the damage. *Lansing* himself is partly responsible for this misconception. He wrote in one of his papers: 'In the early-born lines, longevity increased slowly but steadily through successive generations ... On the other hand, in the late-born lines, longevity was shortened in each successive generation with final extinction of the line ... it appeared that the eggs of adult rotifers transmit a capacity to accelerate ageing which is cumulative ... This capacity is not expressed by eggs from adolescent mothers' (*Lansing,* 1956). These conclusions contain both overstatements and understatements. It is worthwhile to have a closer look at some of his experiments.

Rotifers, or Rotatoria, are microscopic fresh water organisms. Their size is small and it varies from 0.25 to 1 mm in length. However, within this minute body a great variety of organs is contained. In the two species used by *Lansing,* only female parthenogenetic eggs are laid which hatch in about 24 h. After a period of immaturity which varies with the species, the rotifer lays eggs at the rate of one to five per day. *P. citrina* lives for about 20 days and lays an average of 23 eggs during this period. *E. triquetra* lives approximately for 8 days and lays only about 10 eggs.

In a first experiment, *Lansing* bred orthoclones of *P. citrina* at 4, 11 and 17 days for 4, 3 and 2 generations, respectively. In the young orthoclone, no significant change in total egg production was noticeable. However, the fecundity of his middle-aged and old orthoclones dropped consistently in the last two generations of the 11-day orthoclone, F_2 and F_3, and in the last generation of the 17-day orthoclone. In a second experiment, 5-, 11- and 16-day orthoclones were followed for 7, 4 and 2 generations. Both total egg production and longevity remained constant throughout the experiment. In a third experiment, 8- and 17-day orthoclones were followed for 7 and 2 generations. Total egg production declined in the last generation only. Thus, the decrease in fecundity is in general apparent only in the last living generation, the other having a relatively constant egg production. More important, however, is the fact — which, for some obscure reason, has been overlooked by all reviewers, including myself (*Lints and Hoste*, 1974) — that *all* of Lansing's orthoclones, including the orthoclones bred from young parents, died out after a certain number of generations. They became extinct because the eggs laid either did not develop or were inadequate in number, or because the females became totally sterile.

In 1948, *Lansing* made some supplementary experiments, with 7- and 6-day orthoclones which again died out after 15 and 17 generations, respectively. Extinction of the orthoclones was due, as previously, to a drastic reduction either in fecundity or in fertility.

Lansing then claimed that the 'ageing factor', the accumulation of which he believed was the reason for the extinction of an orthoclone, started to appear in *P. citrina* around the time of cessation of growth, i.e. around the fifth or sixth day of life. He also assumed that there is an inverse relationship between the age at which successive generations are reproduced and the longevity of the orthoclones (*Lansing*, 1956). However, when the complete data of both 1947 and 1948 are considered, the postulated quasi-linear relationship disappears (fig. 22). Clearly, in *P. citrina*, continuous reproduction at a fixed age has detrimental effects on the offspring, *whatever the age of reproduction*, the worst periods being at the beginning and at the end of the life cycle, the least bad being at middle age. The original idea of *Lansing* who claimed that the death of his orthoclones was due to a 'transmissible and cumulative *ageing* factor' must, we believe, be replaced by the idea of a 'transmissible and cumulative *age* factor'.

In a last series of experiments, *Lansing* was able to show that the extinction of his old orthoclones could be prevented, at least temporarily! He obtained this

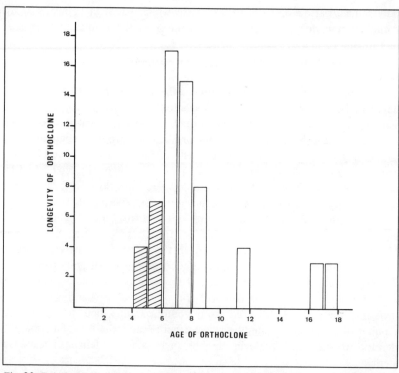

Fig. 22. Relation between the longevity, in generations, and the age at reproduction, in days, of an orthoclone in *P. citrina*. Irrespective of the age of reproduction, the constant reproduction at a fixed age has cumulative detrimental effects on the offspring, which culminate, sooner or later, in the extinction of the orthoclone. Drawn, with permission from (hatched columns) tables I and II in *Lansing* (1947) and from (blanc columns) figure 6 in *Lansing* (1948).

result when, after a certain number of generations of reproduction at an old age, the 11- and 16-day orthoclones were no longer reproduced at 11 or 16 days but at 5 days instead. From this, he deduced that the transmissible and cumulative age factor was also reversible and thus extragenic.

b. Lansing Effects of Other Organisms

These results have been confirmed, more or less clearly – in a way depending essentially on the rigour of the experimental conditions and on the patience of the experimentor – in various species, mainly insects: in *D. melanogaster* (*David*, 1961; *O'Brian*, 1961), in *D. pseudoobscura* (*Wattiaux*, 1968a), in *D. subobscura* (*Wattiaux*, 1968b), in *Tenebrio molitor* (*Ludwig and Fiore*,

1960), in *T. castaneum* (*Sokal,* 1970; *Mertz,* 1975), in *Musca domestica* (*Callahan,* 1962), in *Caenorhabditis elegans* (*Beguet,* 1972). More data and critical reviews in *Lints and Hoste* (1974, 1977).

In mammals, the studies on the influence of continuous reproduction at a given age has been made only on mice, mostly inbred lines, by *Strong* and his co-workers (review in *Strong,* 1968). They showed the influence of both the maternal age and of the age of the orthoclone. For instance, the female F_1 offspring of a group of mice aged 201–300 days have mammary gland tumours later in life and, when free of tumours, live longer than female mice born from females either younger or older than 201–300 days. Even more interesting is the fact that the onset of lung tumours in mice derived from a 201- to 300-day orthoclone is later in life than in offspring of both younger and older orthoclones. The influence of continuous reproduction at a fixed age was also shown on such traits as age at first litter, appearance of fibro-sarcomas after the injection of a chemical carcinogen, longevity and so on.

Repeated reproduction at young or old age has even effects on behavioural traits. *Elens et al.* (1966) created, among a non-inbred stock of albino mice, a young orthoclone by reproduction, for twelve generations, through young females of less than 3 months, and an old orthoclone by reproduction, for three generations, through 'old' mothers of more than 12 months. The learning ability of these mice was tested in a double-T Vicari's maze to determine how effectively fasted members of young and old orthoclones would learn to run through the maze directly to food. The superiority in learning ability of the individuals of the old orthoclone is obvious, although their mean number of errors is greater during their first trials. The individuals from the young orthoclone do not learn at all (fig. 23).

Plant material constitutes a special challenge in the search of parental age or Lansing effects. Indeed, most plants appear to be more or less immortal; senescence and death in monocarpic and short-lived plants are clearly associated with flower or fruit formation. Their limited life-span depends essentially on mechanical factors and on a variety of selective environmental factors (review in *Woolhouse,* 1974). Apical meristems grow continuously and are concomitantly rejuvenated. In this aspect, the experiment of *Ashby and Wangermann* (1954) on the clonally reproducing waterplant *Lemna minor* is particularly interesting.

Lemna minor is a waterplant which reproduces rapidly by vegetative means to give uniform clones. The entire plant body consists of a flattened, roughly elliptical frond, about 10 mm^2 in area and with a single root. Daughter fronds arise on either side of the node, each at first enclosed in its own pocket in the mother frond tissue. Very early in the development of a daughter frond, a knob of meristematic tissue, the next daughter frond, appears to its dorsal side. All this time, a few cells at the base of the frond elongate to many times their original length forming a long stripe which separates the fully grown daughter

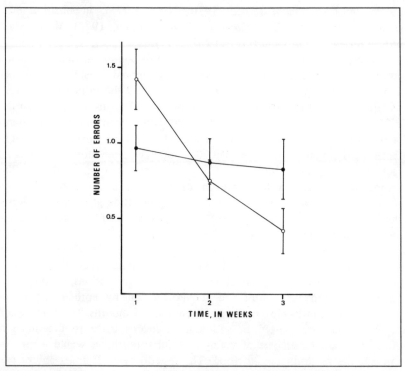

Fig. 23. Learning ability in mice. Mean number of errors, tested in a double-T maze, for members of young (•) and old (○) orthoclones, aged 1 year. The training of the animals lasted 3 weeks, and one trial a day, for 5 days, was given each week. The data for the same week are averaged. The confidence limits for a t = 0.05 are given. Redrawn with permission from *Elens et al.* (1966).

frond from the mother frond. Eventually, the stripe breaks and the first daughter frond begins an independent existence. The breaking away of fully grown daughter fronds results in a constant amount of meristematic and adult tissue in the mother frond throughout its life.

Ashby and Wangermann found that the surface of fully grown successive daughter fronds is inversely proportional to the age of the mother frond. The decrease in surface area is impressive, decreasing from 9.9 mm^2 when the mother frond is 3.5 days to 1.6 mm^2 when it is 60 days (fig. 24). More interesting is the fate of the daughter fronds produced by late daughter fronds: the first of them is larger than the frond from which it is produced. This continues for many generations – up to six for very small late daughter fronds – until the maximum area is restored. Thus, the meristems of the successive daughters of a given frond

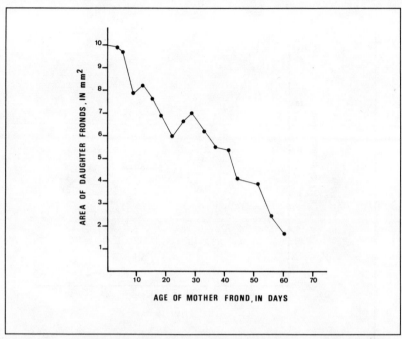

Fig. 24. In *Lemna minor* the areas of successive daughter fronds when fully grown become progressively smaller, the older the mother frond. The first daughter frond produced by a small daughter frond is itself not equally small or smaller but considerably larger than the small frond which produced it. This increase in area of the first daughter frond, compared with its mother frond, continues from generation to generation until maximum area is restored. Drawn with permission from table I in *Ashby and Wangermann* (1954).

age progressively and those from one generation of fronds to the next rejuvenate progressively.

It is evident that the transmission, the cumulation and the progressive reversibility of an extragenic factor influencing growth and ageing depend on age in a non-random way. This is further and clearly ascertained by the fact that any treatment which alters the length of life of the mother fronds also alters the rate of diminution of area from daughter to daughter frond. This is illustrated, for example, by the effects of growing one set of fronds at 20 °C and another at 30 °C. Raising the temperature by 10 °C halves the length of life of the mother fronds and at the same time doubles the rate at which the size of successive daughter fronds diminishes. In the present case, the idea of relative parental age gains credence in a particularly evident way (p. 67).

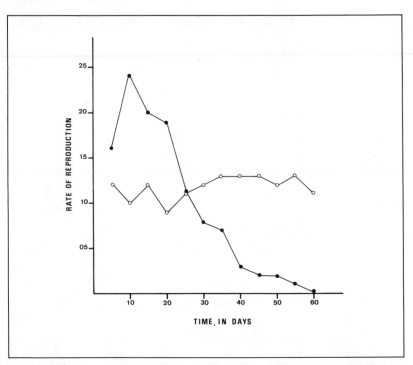

Fig. 25. Rate of reproduction of lines of successive anteriors (●) and of lines of successive posteriors (○) in *S. incaudatum.* The rate of reproduction is expressed in number of divisions per line per day averaged for successive periods of 5 days. 10 lines of successive anteriors and 4 lines of successive posteriors were observed. Redrawn with permission from *Sonneborn* (1930).

An experiment which, *mutatis mutandis,* resembles the preceding one was done by *Sonneborn* (1930) using a turbellarian flatworm, *Stenostomum in-caudatum. S. incaudatum* reproduces asexually by transverse fission. This division separates the individual into two parts, a large anterior portion of 1.15 mm long, and a smaller posterior part of approximately 0.45 mm long. The anterior product has only to regenerate a small tail component while the posterior part has to grow a new trunk and heat. Thus, in the anterior part there is a limited amount of growth activity, while in the posterior part there is an abundance of growth.

Sonneborn created a series of lines of successive anterior individuals on the one hand, and a series of lines of successive posterior individuals, on the other hand. These lines differ in many ways with respect to growth, ageing and life-span. The rate of reproduction in lines of successive anterior individuals is high at first, but gradually declines to zero; in lines of successive posteriors, it is uniformly moderate (fig. 25). All anterior lines invariably die; not all posterior lines die when kept under observation for periods much longer than the mean and as long as the maximum length of life observed among lines of successive anteriors. (Those posterior lines which die appear to do so only as a result of unfavourable environmental conditions.) Growth and life-span appear to be closely linked.

c. Lansing Effects in *Drosophila*

Recently, the Lansing effects were systematically reinvestigated in *D. melanogaster.* A wild strain was bred both at young and old age for ten generations. In each system of reproduction, three replicates were made. Each of these replicates was exposed to a different selection programme, related to abdominal bristle number. The experiments were repeated twice. Longevity and various parameters relating to fecundity were measured. In both experiments, the mean longevity drops regularly — the rates being, however, extremely different and a function of the system of reproduction — to around 40% of the wild strain longevity, increases afterwards up to the original value — again at very different rates — and then remains apparently stable (fig. 26). The same pattern is found for fecundity which decreases first to 20% of the wild strain fecundity, and is afterwards restored to more or less its original value (*Lints and Hoste,* 1974, 1977).

Our results parallel those of *Lansing* on four points. The continuous reproduction from both young and old parents alters fecundity and longevity to a considerable extent. The effects of such systems of reproduction are cumulative; they are reversible; they are due neither to classical genic nor to environmental factors. That the effects are not due to genic variations is suggested by the fact that they appear twice in six lines submitted to very different selection programmes and which therefore diverge genetically as the selection proceeds. It is further suggested by the fact that they are twice reversible in all six lines. That they are not due to uncontrolled environmental variations, the so-called intangible variations, is shown by the regular and evolutive nature of the phenomenon. That they are not due to other environmental influences, linked for instance to climatic or other yearly changes, is suggested by the fact that the maximal and minimal peaks in life-span and fecundity observed in the lines reproduced either at a young or at an old age do not appear at the same calendar time.

Our results differ, or rather are complementary to *Lansing*'s results on two important points. The accumulation of parental age effects does not culminate in the extinction of the lines. The reversibility of the parental age effects is not induced by a change in the age at which reproduction occurs but by a feed-back mechanism present in the strain itself.

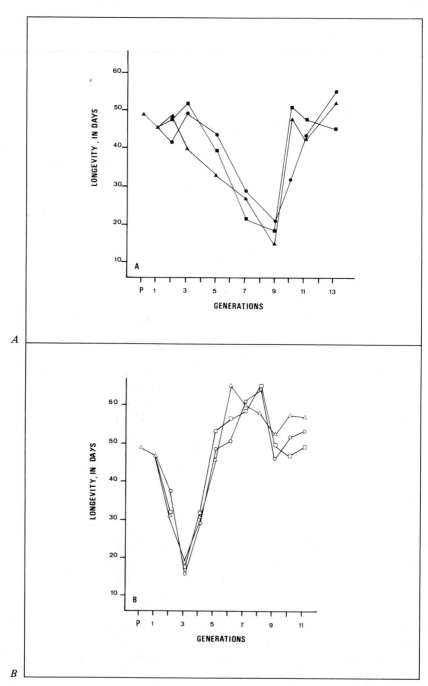

2. The Mechanism of the Lansing Effects

We have seen that with the exception of traits which are directly related to genetic 'accidents' — mutations, chromosomal non-disjunction and so on — the mean expression of most quantitative traits in *Drosophila*, and other organisms, varies in a non-linear way as a function of parental age, showing one or more peaks during the life cycle of the parental individual. This implies that ovogenesis and possibly also spermatogenesis — but on this point the evidence is not convincing — do not produce eggs of a constant 'quality'. This is, however, not surprising: one has only to bear in mind, for instance, the high mortality of eggs laid during the very first or the last days of life of a *Drosophila* female.

a. Morphogens. Positional Information

Does it mean that the cellular composition and/or the molecular configuration, i.e. the cellular organisation of the ovum vary as a function of maternal age? Such variations — at least in the DNA and RNA content of the eggs of young and old *D. melanogaster* females — have been demonstrated by *Tsien and Wattiaux* (1971). But, as suggested by *Britten and Davidson* (1969) or by *Sussman* (1970) the control of the activities of a cell, a tissue or an organism does not necessarily reside in the presence or absence of DNA or any other polynucleotide type molecule. On theoretical as well as on experimental grounds *Crick* (1970), *Lawrence* (1971) and *Lawrence et al.* (1972) have suggested that gradients of different morphogens may result in differential growth during embryogenesis.

The idea of morphogenetic gradients is not a new one. It derives essentially from the concept of positional information, the first tenants of which were *Wilson* (1896) and *Conklin* (1905). The modern version of positional information has been defended by *Davidson* (1968) and particularly by *Wolpert* (1969) (see also *Wolpert and Lewis,* 1975). However, until recently, only very indirect

---

Fig. 26. Variations in the longevity of females in the successive generations of a wild strain of *D. melanogaster* constantly reproduced at young (A) and old (B) age. The *D. melanogaster* strain used was derived from four *Drosophila* wild-type laboratory strains, from various origins, maintained by mass-mating for several years in the laboratory at a constant temperature of 25 °C (*Gruwez et al.,* 1971). A high and a low selection line — for abdominal bristle number — and a control line were reproduced, generation after generation, at a young age, namely 4 days after emergence. Another series of selection and control lines were reproduced at an old age. At the beginning of the experiment, the old age was fixed at 26 days. However, as the experiment proceeded, the fecundity of the successive generations decreased parallel to their longevity, the reproduction age had to be modified and was then defined as the age where 80–90% of the females of all the old orthoclones still laid 20 to 30 fertile eggs a day. In the old orthoclone, the P generation and 11 successive generations were observed; in the young orthoclone, the P and 9 out of 13 successive generations. ● = High line; ▲ = control line; ■ = low line. Redrawn from *Lints and Hoste* (1974).

evidence suggested the existence of such information, linked to specific cyto-plasmic molecules. Such indirect evidence originated, for instance, from the study of insect development. Normally an insect consists of a certain number of segments — each segment being uniquely patterned — arranged in order from head to tail. This order becomes defined in most insect eggs very early during development and more precisely at the blastoderm stage. It depends solely on the position of the cells at the surface of the egg, and not at all on the lineage of their nuclei. The eggs thus contain positional information. The work of *Hotta and Benzer* (1972) on *Drosophila* mosaics is particularly convincing in this respect.

In *Smittia,* a tiny dipteran midge, *Kalthoff* (1971) was able to localize a type of positional information leading, when disturbed, to the formation of a modified segment pattern, the so-called 'double abdomen'. Head, thorax and anterior abdominal segments of that chironomid midge are replaced by an additional set of posterior abdominal segments formed in mirror image sym-metry to the original abdomen. The information relevant to that aberrant pattern is unevenly distributed in the anterior third of the egg, becoming most concentrated at the anterior tip. Recently, some insight into the nature of such information was gained by experiments which produced double abdomens by gently puncturing the anterior pole of the *Smittia* egg in water containing RNase (*Kandler-Singer and Kalthoff,* 1976). Puncturing of eggs elsewhere than at the anterior pole produced no double abdomen. Furthermore, double abdomens were formed only when the experiment was performed up to the blastoderm stage of embryogenesis. According to *Lawrence* (1976), these results strongly suggest that a fraction of RNA is an essential component in the generation of positional information in the egg. We guess that these results may be put side by side with those of *Tsien and Wattiaux* (1971) who showed, as we have seen, that the RNA content of the egg of *D. melanogaster* varies as a function of maternal age.

In *D. melanogaster, Bull* (1966) studied an inherited lethal disturbance in egg polarity, the so-called bicaudal which, no doubt, resembles the double abdomen syndrome in *Smittia.* The bicaudal abnormal embryos develop the terminal segments of a second larval abdomen in mirror image symmetry to the terminal segments of the normal abdomen. The interest of bicaudal — which is produced in very low frequency — stems from two facts. Firstly, the production of these lethal disturbances is associated with an unmarked second chromosome which has been carried in three separate inbred lines in combination with a Curly, Lobe, speck balance stock. Secondly, reciprocal crosses of flies capable of producing the syndrome with flies unable to do so have shown that the maternal genotype is the controlling factor in the production of the abnormality.

Bull considers various hypotheses. For instance, he holds that information programming the embryonic axis is stored in the cortex of the egg cytoplasm during oogenesis, or that genes in the nurse cells control oocyte differentiation, or that the activity of the genes is very sensitive to the internal maternal environment.

b. 'Molecular Geography'

The hypotheses of *Bull* give some ground to the model of *Davidson and Britten* (1971) concerning the control of gene expression during development. The model assumes that there exists an initial divergence in genetic activity due to an unequal distribution of egg cytoplasmic regulatory elements among the different cells in early cleavage. *Davidson and Britten* (see also *Krause and Sander,* 1962) suppose that the major part of the regulation of genetic activity probably occurs at the level of transcriptional control through some sensor structures (genes) sensible to sensor proteins stored from oogenesis in the cortical particles of the egg.

Such a non-homogeneous distribution of molecules has been shown in the *Drosophila* egg cytoplasm. *Graziosi and Roberts* (1975) have indeed shown that some antigens are unequally distributed in the *Drosophila* egg, which suggests that genes are not only regulated in time but also in space. Such could be the underlying mechanism of the nuclear differentiation in ciliates, for instance. The baffling phenomenon of nuclear differentiation within a single cytoplasmic compartment occurs in many animal and plant cell types. In most ciliates, nuclear differentiation occurs during the formation of micro- and macronuclei from a single zygote nucleus during sexual reproduction. The two types of nuclei, which differ strikingly in morphology and nucleic acid content, develop in different regions of the cell. The experiments with *Stentor* (*de Terra,* 1975) show clearly that identical nuclei, sharing a common cytoplasm, can be made grossly asynchronous with regard to morphology and DNA synthesis if they are associated with separate regions of cell surface.

However, these types of information linked in one way or another to genic actions or to the products of gene action should in no way be considered as the sole mechanism of control of differentiation and development. Cytoplasmic organization, 'specific preformed organization of the cells or its parts', 'molecular geography' as *Sonneborn* (1963, 1970) calls it, could be as important for development as any other product of gene action. In a remarkable series of experiments with the unicellular ciliated protozoan *P. aurelia, Beisson and Sonneborn* (1965) have shown that preformed cell structures play a critical role in cell heredity.

P. aurelia is a large unicellular organism. Its cortex is subdivided into longitudinal rows of unit territories bounded by ridges. Unit territories contain one or two cilia and basal bodies positioned in such a way that the examination of any unit territory *in situ* reveals without ambiguity the cell's right, left, anterior and posterior parts. During the minutes preceding cell division the number of unit territories doubles, cilia and basal bodies appearing at a definite place and in a definite orientation (fig. 27) (for full details, see *Dippel*, 1968).

Beisson and Sonneborn (1965) rotated a small patch of unit territories by 180°. They asked whether, if the inverted units reproduced, their parts would show normal or inverted positions and orientations. The result of their research was unambiguous. The *Paramecium* clones obtained by rotation of some unit territories reproduced true to type through hundreds of fissions — in some cases, progeny were followed up to 800 cell generations! — dozens of autogamies and conjugation with normals, with or without endoplasmic exchanges. Never could an exception be found to the rule that when inverted unit territories reproduce their descendant, unit territories are also inverted.

Says *Sonneborn* (1970): 'There is no escape from the conclusion that the site of initiation of basal body assembly, its path of migration to the surface of the cell, and the orientation of associated structures around it are indeed determined by the molecular geography *within* the unit territory and *not* by any other outside influence, either nuclear or cellular.'

Broadly speaking, it appears that various developmental and genetic events which are regionally localized in various parts of the cell may depend upon specific molecular combinations between newly formed molecules deriving from genes and pre-existing molecular patterns already present in the cell.

The fact that nutritional conditions may interfere with the apparition and the modulation of the Lansing effects is a strong argument in favour of the role of cellular composition of the ovum in the expression of various characters of the offspring, such as those discovered in the study of cumulation of parental age effects.

Lansing effects have been shown in the parthenogenetic crustacean *Moina macrocopa* cultured monoxenically on *Chlamydomonas reinhardii*. Though these effects are apparent only when reproduction occurs through successive generations of old mothers, it is not critical to the present discussion. What is important is that these effects can be modified and partly prevented by exposing the animals to inositol or liver infusion (*Murphy and Davidoff*, 1972).

Fig. 27. A Silver impregnation of part of dorsal surface of *P. aurelia,* viewed from the outside. The silvered (black) structures are: the bounding ridges of the unit territory (outlined at u); the puncture of cilia (c) with their basal bodies; the tip of trichocysts (t) in cross-ridges of unit territories. *B* Silver impregnation of *P. aurelia* after amputation of posterior third of body; ventral surface, boundaries of unit territories not silvered. b = 'bald' area free of cilia and basal bodies; v = vestibule, i.e. entrance to ingestatory apparatus. *C* Diagram of part of two normally oriented rows of unit territories (1 and 3) flanking a single row (2) that is rotated by 180°. R = Right; A = anterior; f = kinetodesmal fibre; s = sac; bb = basal bodies. *D* Silver preparation showing two inverted rows of unit territories (2 and 3) flanked by normal rows (1 and 4). Note that sacs (s) are on the 'wrong' side of basal bodies (bb) in rows 2 and 3. With permission from *Sonneborn* (1970).

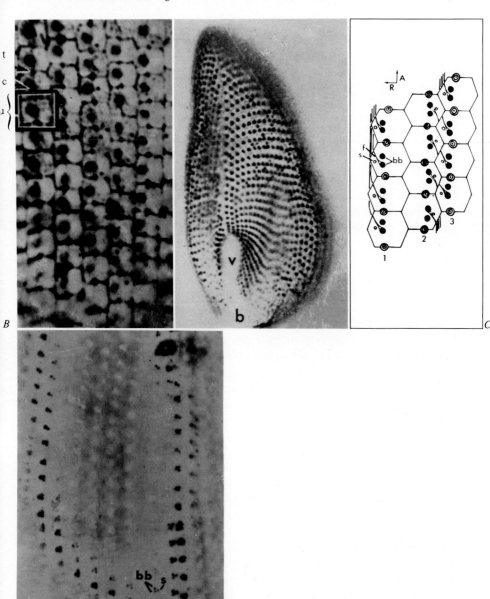

More generally, as initially demonstrated by *Gurdon* and his school (*Gurdon and Brown,* 1965; review in *Gurdon,* 1976), a nucleus from a cell of a given type introduced in the cytoplasm of a cell of another type fails to direct the synthesis of products which it formerly controlled; it will start synthesizing what the actual state of the cytoplasm implies instead.

c. Differential Gametogenesis

Now if, as *Muller* (1963) has argued, differentiation, ageing, senescence and death are various stages of a single process of development, it is logical to admit that specific molecules control these various aspects of development. The 'information' related to such aspects of development must be transmitted from one generation to the other through the ovum and may vary with parental age. In other words, some constituents of the successively laid eggs may vary as a function of ageing in a linear or cyclic way; differentiation and ageing being sequential and coordinated the original constitution of an egg may influence the development and life-span of the individual which will emerge from it as well as the precocious or late apparition of given molecules in the eggs produced by that individual.

That there are variations in the 'informational content' of the ovules as a function of parental age is plausible but not easy to demonstrate from the existing evidence. Curiously enough, almost no qualitative analysis of ovules of females of different ages are available. We already quoted the exceptional work of *Tsien and Wattiaux* (1971). In *D. melanogaster,* they have shown that the DNA content of virgin eggs of middle-aged flies is significantly lower than that of the eggs from young or old female flies. On the contrary, they have observed that the RNA content of eggs of young and old flies is smaller compared to that of the eggs of middle-aged flies.

There is also some indirect evidence. In *Oncopeltus fasciatus,* the milkweed bug, *Richards and Kolderie* (1957) have shown that the first several batches of eggs are relatively light. Average weight then increases to reach a maximum in the period where maximum number of eggs are produced. Subsequent egg weights then drop, but not regularly in the last 30 days of life. (*O. fasciatus* lives for a period of 45–55 days). Terminal batches have a very low weight, about 40% lower than the maximum value. Hatchability of the eggs shows differences somewhat paralleling to the weight differences. Similarly, the rate of development is slower for eggs from the first and last parts of the fecund period. According to *Richards and Kolderie:* 'This quantitative difference implies a qualitative difference in the eggs that can hardly be just a matter of weight and amount of stored reserves.'

In *D. melanogaster, Delcour* (1969) analyzed successive daily batches of eggs. Both egg length and duration of embryonic development show the same convex pattern of variation with parental age, whilst total duration of development varies cyclically with parental age. Further evidence of the same type, mostly in insects, and exclusively related to quantitative differences has been repeatedly reported (reviews in *Delcour,* 1969; *Lints,* 1971; *Lints and Hoste,* 1977; see also p. 61). In a study of oxygen consumption during development of the egg in various genotypes of *D. melanogaster,* it was shown that for certain genotypes there is a positive correlation between total oxygen consumption during embryogenesis – from the moment of egg-laying up to the time of emergence of the larva – and maternal age (*Lints et al.,* 1967).

d. Cumulation in the Lansing Effects

One may thus safely assume that the age of the female has an influence on various quantitative and, most probably, qualitative characters of the ovules. These in turn may explain parental age effects. However, Lansing effects are transmissible and cumulative parental age effects. Therefore, one may wonder how physiological and morphological alterations of an organism, due to the age of its parents, will be transmitted to the next generation. In other words, one has not only to understand how the information linked to parental age is transmitted from one generation to the other but how it is accumulated during several generations. A last point will then concern the mechanism of the eventual reversibility of such accumulation, the Lansing effects appearing to be reversible in some cases.

Clearly one of the factors which, at least among insects, usually varies with parental age is the duration of development (*Richards and Kolderie,* 1957; *Tracey,* 1958; *Ludwig and Fiore,* 1960, 1961; *David,* 1961; *Van Horn,* 1966; *Delcour,* 1969; *Lints and Hoste,* 1977). No doubt that the quality of the egg is involved in such variations. In *D. melanogaster,* duration of development is linked, in a way which remains uncertain, to various quantitative traits such as bristle number (*Wattiaux,* 1962), thoracic size (*Lints,* 1963), adult weight (*Bakker and Nelissen,* 1963), life-span (*Lints and Lints,* 1971a–c; *Lints and Soliman,* 1977) and so on.

In a study of the duration of development in *D. melanogaster, Lints and Gruwez* (1972) have shown that the fluctuations in the duration of development are, for a given generation, determined by the duration of development of the parental generation. During the experiment, all environmental factors known to influence duration of development in one respect or other were defined, controlled and kept as constant as possible. Major fluctuations in the duration of development of about 48 h were observed. (At 22 °C, *D. melanogaster* develops in approximately 12 days.) The large fluctuations in a given generation are found not to be random but to depend, in a precise manner, on the relative duration of development of the preceding generation.

Furthermore and essentially, duration of development has immediate effects on growth rate which is a parameter involving both adult size and duration of development. We have seen in detail (p. 45) the important effects of growth rate on life-span, both in poecilotherms and in homeotherms. However, in the present respect, one should know the extent to which growth rate may modify the molecular composition and configuration, the so-called 'molecular geography' of a developing organism. In an interesting study of temperature effects on day-old pupae in *D. melanogaster, Milkman* (1962, 1967) studied the formation and disturbances of the formation of the wing posterior crossvein. He showed, for instance, that closely controlled temperature shocks applied at one time of the development resulted in precise quantitative and qualitative disturbances in the posterior crossvein formation. Naturally, the sensitive periods are earlier for flies raised at higher temperatures – their development being faster – and later for those raised at lower temperatures. What is striking, however, is the fact that the temperature at which the animals are raised, and which of course considerably modifies their growth rate, has a profound effect on the response to treatment not only quantitatively but also qualitatively. *Milkman* suggests that these differences in adaptation to temperature result from the modifications both in the tertiary and quaternary structures of proteins.

Experiments made with bacteria suggest that growth rate may not only affect the molecular conformation but also the relative molecular composition of a developing organism. In *Escherichia coli, Deusser and Wittmann* (1972) studied the protein composition of the ribosomes as a function of growth rate. Growth rate was modified by growing bacteria in more or less rich media. Each ribosomal protein was analyzed; and the ratio of the relative abundance of the protein in the rich medium to that in the minimal medium was calculated. The proteins could be grouped into four classes with respect to their ratios. About two thirds of all proteins gave ratios between 0.90 and 1.10. A rather large group (S1, S10, S11, S19, S20 from 30S subunits and L8 + L9, L17, L27, L32 and L33 from 50S subunits) has ratios slightly different from those of the first group, but not always reproducible. For proteins L7 and L16, the ratios were 0.8. The ratios for three proteins, whose important functions in the ribosomes are known, namely 3.1 for protein L12, 2.5 for S6 and 2.4 for S2, differ considerably from all others. In *Salmonella typhimurium, Schaechter et al.* (1958) systematically inquired on the size and composition of the cells in steady-state cultures. They demonstrated a strong dependence of mean cell mass on the specific growth rate when growth rate was varied by nutrition, but none when it was varied by temperature.

Growth rate may be defined as the speed at which a series of sequential processes and coordinated interactions give rise to a more or less well balanced organism. In other words, an organism of a given size which is born or emerges after a certain time may be considered as the net result of a series of more or less coordinated, yet conflicting, anabolic and catabolic reactions. For instance, in their work with different species or interspecific hybrids of *Salmo, Gray* (1929)

and *Spaas and Heuts* (1958) have shown that eggs developing at low temperatures result in larger alevins than those developing at high temperatures. Since
the food reserves present in the egg are identical, the observed variations in size
must be attributed to the changing balance between anabolism and catabolism.
In *D. melanogaster* (*Lints and Lints,* 1969, 1971b), the imaginal size and the
duration of development are positively or negatively correlated, depending on
external factors, as temperature or larval crowding. It is then evident that
variations in the speed of overall metabolic processes cannot be due to equal and
parallel variations of the totality of the anabolic and catabolic reactions leading
to the developed organism. In other words, depending on growth rate, diverse
anabolic and catabolic processes may have relative speeds which are entirely
different. They may result in cellular constituents being synthesized either in
larger quantities or earlier than other constituents under one set of conditions,
and either in smaller quantities or later in other conditions. The cellular composition and the configuration of the diverse constitution of the cell may,
therefore, be a function of the relative speeds of the anabolic and catabolic
processes.

In summary, the cumulation of parental age effects may be explained in the
following way. The 'information' related to parental age effects must be transmitted from one generation to the other through the ovule and must be different
as a function of parental age. In other words, some constituents of the successively laid eggs may vary in a linear or cyclic way as a function of ageing;
differentiation and ageing being sequential and coordinated, the original constitution of an egg may influence the development and life-span of the individual
which will emerge from it as well as the precocious or late apparition of
molecules in the eggs that this individual will produce.

e. Reversibility in the Lansing Effects

The spontaneous reversibility of Lansing effects implies that the 'quality' of
the eggs laid generation after generation at a non-optimal age is restored after a
certain number of generations by a kind of feedback mechanism.

More or less spontaneous mechanisms of re-equilibration, with or without
changes in the breeding system, are not entirely unknown. As we have seen, they
have been described in *Aspergillus nidulans* by *Jinks* (1954), in *A. glaucus* by
Mather and Jinks (1958), in *Lemna minor* by *Ashby and Wangermann* (1954), in
D. melanogaster by *Lints and Gruwez* (1972) and *Lints and Hoste* (1977) and of
course by *Lansing* (1947, 1948). Such spontaneous re-equilibration mechanisms
can be explained by assuming that the quality of an egg depends not so much on
the absolute age of the female as on its relative position during ovogenesis.
Indeed, when breeding is carried on successively by young parents, the day of
maximal egg production is situated nearer and nearer to the beginning of the
egg-laying period. In such lines, the eggs used for reproduction become relatively

older in a progressive manner. On the contrary, in the lines reproduced at an old age, the day of maximal egg production is situated later and later in life; the eggs used for reproduction become thus relatively younger progressively (*Lints and Hoste,* 1977). This is not an entirely unknown phenomenon. In mice, *Johnson and Strong* (1963) noticed that inbred lines reproduced during 15 generations at young age had their first litter significantly later in life than lines reproduced during the same number of generations at old age. The existence of a compensatory mechanism similar to the one found in *Drosophila* is evident.

The mechanism of such a progressive feedback phenomenon remains obscure. Yet the first model which comes to mind is the *Delbrück*'s model for alternative steady state of the cytoplasm (*Delbrück,* 1949). This model postulates that some cytoplasmic controlling states are persistent, although reversible. The persistency of such a system is due to a self-perpetuating chain of reactions inhibiting the release of a second chain, responsible for a different cytoplasmic state. The reversibility is due to a change of concentration in one of the inhibiting products of the first chain, due for instance to the environment, which allows the alternative reaction chain to begin to operate.

IV. Conclusion

The study of ageing and death is undoubtedly not a simple one. Ageing is a normal phenomenon; however, the moment of apparition of its first symptoms and the rate at which it progresses are under the influence of a great number of modifying agents, of factors of the environment, in the largest sense of the word.

Maybe was it never enough stressed on the difference which may exist between the moment of death as it is observed and the ideal moment, representative of the potential duration of life. The time of death as it is observed in nature or in the laboratory may be the moment of the end of the potential duration of life, but it may also be due to accidents, to infectious agents, to insufficient or badly balanced nutrition, to the innumerable stresses to which living beings are submitted. On the contrary, the potential duration of life is the one due to the mechanisms intrinsic to a particular organism, defined and programmed by its genotype, and which trigger the onset and control the evolution of senescence. No doubt that discrimination between real and potential life-span exists. The study of *Ross et al.* (1976) (p. 48; tables XIII, XIV) has clearly demonstrated that the individual duration of life of rats could be forecasted — within the limits of a conditional multiple regression analysis — from a series of parameters measured in the early part of the life of animals. These parameters depend either on dietary factors or on growth components. However, what we feel essential in the present respect — i.e. the discrimination between real and potential life-span — is that the predictive capability of the multiple regression equation is improved parallel to the progressive elimination of the shortest-lived individuals.

A second interesting point of this study resides in the fact that the life-span of the longest-lived animals appears to depend exclusively on growth components and not at all on dietary factors. What seems evident from the present review is that ageing and death, like development and differentiation, are genetically controlled, although for the time being the amount of control and the manner in which that control is exerted (*von Hahn,* 1969; *Medvedev,* 1972) remain unanswered problems. We reviewed some direct and indirect evidence in favour of this assertion. Direct proofs related for instance to genetic manipulations such as inbreeding or crossbreeding; we noticed that demonstrations based on genealogical records and on heritability studies had to be considered with some caution.

Nor is the indirect evidence missing. The relation among growth rate, as well as other related parameters, and ageing and death, the rare examples of programmed cell death, and the important but generally ignored influence of parental age on the phenotypic expression of various traits (including longevity) of the progeny, appears to us as essential elements which cannot be neglected or underestimated.

Furthermore, the nature of the Lansing effects and more precisely the fact that they are transmissible, cumulative and reversible does certainly not constitute, as we have seen, an argument in favour of the mutation or derived theories of ageing. On the contrary, the Lansing effects imply that the observed variations are due to some non-permanent modifications in the information-bearing, control or lecture systems. These modifications do not appear to be stochastic; they rather appear to be sequential and coordinated events.

The overall picture which emerges from the whole of the evidence reviewed is that programming occurs through a subtle interaction between gene products and extra-nuclear factors, including cellular composition, configuration and localization. The influence of extra-nuclear factors is particularly obvious in the problem of parental age effects. There is a sort of unfaithful, or rather non-constant, transmission of information from parent to offspring, which is clearly related to parental age and probably programmed. Parental age must obviously be considered as a part of the environment which shapes the phenotype of an individual.

A precise knowledge in molecular terms of what ageing is and how and to what an extent it is controlled by genotype or environment is still missing. Considerable efforts are being made to solve these problems through the analysis of ageing and dying cell strains in culture. It is by no means evident that this will give the clue to the problem. To be sure, there are major changes which occur in ageing cells. Are these major changes causes or effects of ageing? This remains unknown. There are also cells which have a limited life-potential in culture. Does this limited life-potential *in vitro* have any relation with a possible life-potential *in vivo* or even with the normal life-span of a given species? This too remains unknown. Some serious doubts about it have recently been raised by *Macieira-Coelho* (1976). He finds no obvious correlation between cellular life-span *in vitro* and the life-span of the organism itself. This conclusion is based on a few species. The analysis of more cell types is necessary.

As long as ageing and death of cells must be further analyzed, the *in vivo* and *in vitro* fate of particular cell types should be studied and compared. Refined analysis of transformation and reversion is also badly needed. Cells removed from their normal environment may live and die in a way that is only vaguely related to the way they live and die *in vivo*.

Immediate and remote extracellular environment could be of paramount importance in the differentiation and ageing of cells, tissues, organs and so on as argued by different authors in their argument for the morphogens. The studies and the precise definition of the 'carriers of determination' made by the school of *Hadorn* through the elegant analysis of the programmation of isolated determined cells of the imaginal discs of *Drosophila* (reviews in *Gehring and Nöthiger,* 1973; *Gehring,* 1976) is likely to be of great help.

In fact, studies pertaining to ageing cells may certainly yield a great deal of information about cellular senescence and death. It is by no means obvious that they will give the clue to the problem of ageing in organisms. As a matter of fact, these very simple principles, which should be familiar to all biologists, namely that a tissue is not s sum of cells or that an organism is not a sum of organs made out of cells, have probably been too much neglected. The different levels of organization of the living world have their own laws which transcend the laws of the lower levels.

We guess that gerontologists should return, at least partially, to an *in toto* approach of the gerontological problems. Gerontology is of course a young science which evolves slowly and sometimes erratically. It is even by no means evident that the relevant questions have been asked. We do not resist the pleasure of quoting *Sacher,* whose ideas of 1968, in our opinion, remain perfectly sound today. Says *Sacher:* 'Gerontology is a young discipline, and most of its growth occurred within the period of ascendancy of the molecular paradigm. The consequences are obvious, for biological gerontology is regarded by the great majority of its practitioners and expositors as a branch of molecular biology. This is shown only by explicit affirmations, but more convincingly by the unanimity with which experiment protocols conform to the molecular paradigm ... This is an unfortunate misalliance, which could have consequences for gerontology in this century even more disastrous than the misdirection suffered by the social sciences in the nineteenth ... The argument rests on three main points. First, the attempts to produce molecular theories of ageing without reference to any other level of biological phenomena lead to logical fallacies. Second, the molecular view leads to a persistent under-emphasis of certain systemic aspects of ageing and death, to the detriment of progress. Third, a complete and self-sufficient discipline of gerontology can be founded if and only if gerontologists can learn to put the molecular viewpoint back into a correct biological perspective, in which the systemic aspects of the organism are seen to be in some respects more basic than the molecular.'

In this respect, the search for mutants affecting one or the other component of growth and the study of the way these mutants age and die could be extremely interesting as it could show how far death constitutes the last step in development. Experiments of selection for longer and shorter life-spans — experiments which undoubtedly will be technically and financially difficult and which are unfortunately totally inexistent — are also badly needed.

In the present respect, a last word could be said about the evolutionary theory of senescence as well as on the experimental approach to this problem. Remarkably defined by *Medawar* (1952), the theory sounds as follows: 'If hereditary factors achieve their overt expression at some intermediate age of life; if the age of overt expression is variable; and if these variations are themselves inheritable; then natural selection will so act as to enforce the postponement of the age of the expression of those factors that are unfavourable and, correspondingly, to expedite the effects of those that are favourable ...' Invoking, in general terms, the possible influence of pleiotropy and linkage, the determinism of such recession or precession of the variable age-effects of genes is not clearly defined in *Medawar*'s paper, whose purpose was, however, not the modelling of such a mechanism.

Several authors have reformulated and sometimes refined *Medawar*'s theory of senescence. *Williams* (1957) suggests that senescence could have evolved by selection of genes that have different effects on fitness at different ages, and more precisely of pleiotropic genes with beneficial effects in the first stages of life history and with deleterious effects in later life. *Edney and Gill* (1968) suppose that the hazard factor, i.e. chances of accidental death, added to the effects of extrinsically caused senescence, including mechanical wear, sets a specific limit to the longevity of a given species, with the consequence that a load of deleterious random mutations and gene interactions, applicable only in later life, would be allowed to accumulate, permitting intrinsic senescence to develop. *Guthrie* (1969) supposes some genes to affect the way in which energy is used for development, reproduction, and so on. In his view, senescence would be the result of energy exhaustion and the adaptative evolution of senescence would depend on a rather unclearly defined balance of selection pressures acting both to decrease and to increase the expression of senescence, the equilibrium point and the strength of the stabilizing pressures being determined by the particular ecological situation of the species.

The evolutionary theory of senescence was the subject of a rather small number of experimental approaches (*Wattiaux*, 1968a, b; *Sokal*, 1970; *Mertz*, 1975) which, anyhow, remain inconclusive (critical review in *Lints and Hoste*, 1977). These studies are based upon the reproduction at an old age during a certain number of generations and on the observation of the fitness of the resulting individuals. The analysis of the Lansing effects has shown the unsuitability of such an approach. Indeed, it will be extremely difficult, if not impossible, to study the effects of a selection for Medawar's or William's type of genes, as advocated by the tenants of the evolutionary theory of ageing, independently from the effects of parental age and, anyhow, before the determinism of these effects is really understood. This is not so.

Another approach could be tried. Ecological divergence, which is due to an adaptation to a variety of ecological niches and which may mimic to a certain extent evolutionary divergence, should be studied in different species. Variations in fitness, in growth components, in ageing and longevity, the relationship between the variations observed should be thoroughly analyzed in the largest possible array of biotopes.

For a long time evolution, this marvellous phenomenon, has been — and still is — thought to depend mainly on a randomly acting factor, i.e. mutation. Today, considering the numerous culs-de-sac into which the reverence for the dogma has led, some start to question explicitely the theory (*Grasse*, 1973; *Løvtrup*, 1977). Ageing theories have not yet the weight nor the *vis inertiae* of a dogma. The evidence here collected leads us to think that ageing and death are not random events, but on the contrary the ultimate steps of this other marvellous phenomenon, namely the development of a living being. Let us hope that the consideration of this evidence may help somewhat to close one or the other blind alley.

V. References

Anonymous: How many globin genes? Nature, Lond. *236:* 10–11 (1972).

Ashby, E. and Wangermann, E.: The effects of meristem aging on the morphology and behavior of fronds in *Lemna minor.* Ann. N.Y. Acad. Sci. *57:* 476–483 (1954).

Baird, M.B.; Samis, H.V.; Massie, H.R., and Zimmerman, J.A.: A brief argument in opposition to Orgel hypothesis. Gerontologia *21:* 57–63 (1975).

Bakker, K. and Nelissen, F.X.: On the relations between the duration of the larval and pupal period, weight and diurnal rhythm in emergence in *Drosophila melanogaster.* Entomol. exp. appl. *6:* 37–52 (1963).

Beardmore, J.A.; Lints, F.A., and Al-Baldawi, A.L.F.: Parental age and heritability of sternopleural chaeta number in *Drosophila melanogaster.* Heredity *34:* 71–82 (1975).

Beardmore, J.A. and Shami, S.A.: Parental age, genetic variation and selection; in *Karlin and Nevo* Population genetics and ecology, pp. 3–22 (Academic Press, New York 1976).

Beeton, M. and Pearson, K.: Data for the problem of evolution in man. III. A first study of the inheritance of longevity and the selective death-rate in man. Proc. R. Soc. *65:* 290–305 (1899).

Beeton, M. and Pearson, K.: On the inheritance of the duration of life and on the intensity of natural selection in man. Biometrika *1:* 50–89 (1901).

Beguet, B.: The persistence of processes regulating the level of reproduction in the hermaphrodite nematode *Caenorhabditis elegans,* despite the influence of parental aging, over several consecutive generations. Expl Gerontol. *7:* 207–218 (1972).

Beisson, J. and Sonneborn, T.M.: Cytoplasmic inheritance of the organization of the cell cortex in *Paramecium aurelia.* Proc. natn. Acad. Sci. USA *53:* 275–282 (1965).

Bell, A.G.: The duration of life and conditions associated with longevity. A study of the Hyde genealogy (Genealogical Records Office, Washington 1918).

Benedict, W.F.; Jones, P.A.; Lang, W.E.; Igel, H.J., and Freeman, A.E.: Characterization of human cells transformed *in vitro* by urethane. Nature, Lond. *256:* 322–324 (1975).

Benjamin, B.: Actuarial aspects of human lifespans. Ciba Found. Coll. on Ageing, 1959, vol. 5, pp. 2–20.

Berger, S. and Schweiger, H.G.: Fine structural changes of the cell nucleus after implantation into a cytoplasm of a different developmental stage. Proc. 2nd Eur. Symp. Cell Cycle, 1973, pp. 49–50.

Berger, S. and Schweiger, H.G.: Cytoplasmic induction of changes in the ultrastructure of the *Acetabularia* nucleus and perinuclear cytoplasm. J. Cell Sci. *17:* 517–529 (1975).

Bergner, A.D.: The effect of prolongation of each stage of the life-cycle on crossing over in the second and third chromosomes of *Drosophila melanogaster.* J. exp. Zool. *50:* 107–163 (1928).

Biology Data Book. Federation of American Societies for Experimental Biology, Bethesda, Md.; 2nd ed., vol. 2: compiled and edited by *Altman and Dittmer* (1973).

Bishop, J.O.; Pemberton, R., and Baglioni, C.: Reiteration frequency of haemoglobin genes in the duck. Nature new Biol. *235:* 231–234 (1972).

Bodenstein, D.: Factors influencing growth and metamorphosis of the salivary gland in *Drosophila.* Biol. Bull. *84:* 13–33 (1943).

Bodmer, W.F.: Effects of maternal age on the incidence of congenital abnormalities in mouse and man. Nature, Lond. *190:* 1134–1135 (1961).

Bollo, R. and Brot, N.: Age-dependent changes in enzymes involved in macromolecular synthesis in *Turbatrix aceti.* Archs Biochem. Biophys. *164:* 227–236 (1975).

Bootsma, D.; Mulder, M.P.; Pott, F., and Cohen, J.A.: Different inherited levels of DNA repair replication in *Xeroderma pigmentosum* cell strains after exposure to ultraviolet irradiation. Mutat. Res. *9:* 507–516 (1970).

Boveri, T.: Zur Frage der Entstehung maligner Tumoren (Fischer, Jena 1914).

Bozcuk, A.N.: DNA synthesis in the absence of somatic cell division associated with ageing in *Drosophila subobscura.* Expl Gerontol. *7:* 147–156 (1972).

Bozcuk, A.N.: Testing the protein error hypothesis of ageing in *Drosophila.* Expl Gerontol. *11:* 103–112 (1976).

Bridges, C.B.: The relation of the age of the female to crossing over in the third chromosome of *Drosophila melanogaster.* J. gen. Physiol. *8:* 689–700 (1927).

Bridges, C.B.: Variation in crossing over in relation to age of female in *Drosophila melanogaster.* Carneg. Inst. Wash. Publ. *399:* 63–89 (1929).

Britten, R.J. and Davidson, E.H.: Gene regulation for higher cells: a theory. Science, N.Y. *165:* 349–357 (1969).

Brown, D.D. and Dawid, J.B.: Developmental genetics. Annu. Rev. Genet. *3:* 127–154 (1969).

Bull, A.L.: Bicaudal, a genetic factor which affects the polarity of the embryo in *Drosophila melanogaster.* J. exp. Zool. *161:* 221–241 (1966).

Bullough, W.S.: The evolution of differentiation (Academic Press, New York 1967).

Bullough, W.S. and Ebling, F.J.: Cell replacement in the epidermis and sebaceous glands of the mouse. J. Anat. *86:* 29–34 (1952).

Burch, P.R.J. and Jackson, D.: Molecular mechanisms of ageing. A critique. Gerontology *22:* 206–211 (1976).

Burcombe, J.V. and Hollingsworth, M.J.: The relationship between developmental temperature and longevity in *Drosophila.* Gerontologia *16:* 172–181 (1970).

Burnet, F.M.: An immunological approach to ageing. Lancet *ii:* 358–360 (1970).

Burnet, F.M.: Intrinsic mutagenesis. A genetic approach to ageing (MTP, Lancaster 1974).

Caldecott, R.S.: Seedling height, oxygen availability, storage and temperature; their relation to radiation induced genetic injury in barley; in Effects of ionizing radiation on seeds, pp. 3–24 (Int. Atomic Energy Agency, Wien 1961).

Callahan, R.F.: Effects of parental age on the life cycle of the house fly, *Musca domestica* Linnaeus (Diptera: Muscidae). J. N.Y. entomol. Soc. *70:* 150–158 (1962).

Callan, H.G.: The organization of genetic units in chromosomes. J. Cell Sci. *2:* 1–7 (1967).

Carrel, A. and Ebeling, A.H.: Age and multiplication of fibroblasts. J. exp. Med. *34:* 599–623 (1921).

Castor, C.W. and Baker, B.L.: The localisation of adrenocortical steroids on epidermis and connective tissue of the skin. Endocrinology *47:* 234–241 (1950).

Cavalli-Sforza, L.L. and Bodmer, W.F.: The genetics of human populations (Freeman, San Francisco 1971).

Clark, A.M.: Genetic factors associated with ageing; in *Strehler* Adv. Gerontol. Res., vol. 1, pp. 207–255 (Academic Press, New York 1964).

Clark, A.M.; Bertrand, H.A., and Smith, R.E.: Life span differences between haploid and diploid males of *Habrobracon serinopae* after exposure as adults to X-rays. Am. Nat. *97:* 203–208 (1963).

Clark, A.M. and Rockstein, M.: Aging in insects; in *Rockstein* The physiology of insecta, vol. 1, pp. 227–281 (Academic Press, New York 1964).

Clark, A.M. and Rubin, M.A.: The modification by X-irradiation of the life span of haploids and diploids of the wasp, *Habrobracon* sp. Radiat. Res. *15:* 244–253 (1961).

Clarke, J.M. and Maynard Smith, J.: The genetics and cytology of *Drosophila subobscura.* XI. Hybrid vigour and longevity. J. Genet. *53:* 172–180 (1955).

Clarke, J.M. and Maynard Smith, J.: Increase in the rate of protein synthesis with age in *Drosophila subobscura.* Nature, Lond. *209:* 627–629 (1966).

Clarke, R.D.: Proc. Centen Assembl. Inst. Acta *2:* 12 (1950).

Cleaver, J.E.: Repair replication in Chinese hamster cells after damage from ultraviolet light. Photochem. Photobiol. *12:* 17–28 (1970).

Cohen, B.H.: Family patterns of mortality and life span. Q. Rev. Biol. *39:* 130–181 (1964).

Collinge, W.E.: Notes on the terrestrial Isopoda (Woodlice). Northw. Nat. *19:* 112 (1944).

Collins, L.R.: Monotremes and marsupials (Smithsonian, Washington 1973).

Comfort, A.: Longevity and mortality in dogs of four breeds. J. Geront. *15:* 126–129 (1960).

Comfort, A.: A life table for Arabian mares. J. Geront. *17:* 14 (1962).

Comfort, A.: Ageing. The biology of senescence; 2nd ed. (Routledge & Kegan, London 1964).

Comfort, A.: Feasibility in age research. Nature, Lond. *217:* 320–322 (1968).

Conklin, E.G.: The organization and cell-lineage of the ascidian egg. J. Acad. nat. Sci., Philad. *13:* 3–119 (1905).

Crick, F.: Diffusion in embryogenesis. Nature, Lond. *225:* 420–422 (1970).

Cristofalo, V.J. and Kabakjian, J.: Lysosomal enzymes and aging *in vitro:* subcellular enzyme distribution and effect of hydrocortisone on cell life-span. Mech. Age. Dev. *4:* 19–28 (1975).

Crowley, C. and Curtis, H.J.: The development of somatic mutations in mice with age. Proc. natn. Acad. Sci. USA *49:* 626–628 (1963).

Curtis, H.J.: The late effects of radiation. Proc. Am. phil. Soc. *107:* 5–10 (1963).

Curtis, H.J.: Biological mechanisms of aging (Thomas, Springfield 1966).

Curtis, H.J. and Crowley, C.: Chromosome aberrations in liver cells in relation to the somatic mutation theory of aging. Radiat. Res. *19:* 337–344 (1963).

Curtis, H.J. and Gebhard, K.L.: Radiation induced aging in mice. Proc. 2nd Int. Conf. on Peaceful Uses of Atomic Energy, vol. 22, pp. 53–57 (United Nations, Genève 1958).

Curtis, H.J.; Leith, J., and Tilley, J.: Chromosome aberrations in liver cells of dogs of different ages. J. Geront. *21:* 268–270 (1966).

Curtis, H.J. and Miller, K.: Chromosome aberrations in liver cells of guinea pigs. J. Geront. *26:* 292–293 (1971).

Cutler, R.G.: Redundancy of information content in the genome of mammalian species as a protective mechanism determining aging rate. Mech. Age. Dev. *2:* 381–408 (1973/74).

Danes, B.S.: Progeria: a cell culture study on aging. J. clin. Invest. *50:* 2000–2003 (1971).

Daniel, C.W.; Deome, K.B.; Young, J.T.; Blair, P.B., and Faulkin, L.J.: The *in vivo* life span of normal and preneoplastic mouse mammary glands: a serial transplantation study. Proc. natn. Acad. Sci. USA *61:* 53–60 (1968).

Daniel, C.W. and Young, J.T.: Influence of cell division on an aging process. Expl Cell Res. *65:* 27–32 (1971).

Darlington, C.D. and Cour, L. la: The detection of inert genes. J. Hered. *32:* 115–121 (1941).

David, J.: Influence de l'âge de la femelle sur les dimensions des œufs de *Drosophila melanogaster.* C.r. hebd. Séanc. Acad. Sci., Paris *249:* 1145–1147 (1959).

David, J.: Influence de l'état physiologique des parents sur les caractères des descendants. Annls Génét. *3:* 1–78 (1961).

David, J.: Influence de l'âge de la mère sur les dimensions des œufs dans une souche vestigial de *Drosophila melanogaster* Meig. Bull. biol. Fr. Belg. *96:* 505–528 (1962).

Davidson, E.H.: Gene activity in early development (Academic Press, New York 1968).

Davidson, E.H. and Britten, R.J.: Note on the control of gene expression during development. J. theor. Biol. *32:* 123–130 (1971).

Decosse, J.J.; Gossens, C.; Kuzma, J.F., and Unsworth, B.R.: Embryonic inductive tissues that cause histologic differentiation of murine mammary carcinoma *in vitro.* J. natn. Cancer Inst. *54:* 913–922 (1975).

Delbrück, M.: Génétique du bactériophage; in Unités biologiques douées de continuité génétique, pp. 91–103 (Centre national de la recherche scientifique, Paris 1949).

Delcour, J.: Influence de l'âge parental sur la dimension des œufs, la durée de développement et la taille thoracique des descendants chez *Drosophila melanogaster.* J. Insect Physiol. *15:* 1999–2011 (1969).

Delcour, J. and Heuts, M.J.: Cyclic variations in wing size related to parental ageing in *Drosophila melanogaster.* Expl Gerontol. *3:* 45–53 (1968).

Deusser, E. and Wittmann, H.G.: Ribosomal proteins: variation of the protein composition in *Escherichia coli* ribosomes as function of growth rate. Nature, Lond. *238:* 269–270 (1972).

Devi, A.; Lemonde, V.; Srivastava, V. and Sarkar, N.: Nucleic acid and protein metabolism in *Tribolium confusum* Duval. Expl Cell Res. *29:* 443–450 (1963).

Dingley, F. and Maynard Smith, J.: Temperature acclimatization in the absence of protein synthesis in *Drosophila subobscura.* J. Insect Physiol. *14:* 1185–1194 (1968).

Dingley, F. and Maynard Smith, J.: Absence of a life-shortening effect of amino-acid analogues on adult *Drosophila.* Expl Gerontol. *4:* 145–149 (1969).

Dippell, R.V.: The development of basal bodies in *Paramecium.* Proc. natn. Acad. Sci. USA *61:* 461–468 (1968).

Dobzhansky, T. and Wallace, B.: The genetics of homeostasis in *Drosophila.* Proc. natn. Acad. Sci. USA *39:* 162–171 (1953).

Durrant, A.: The environmental induction of heritable change in *Linum.* Heredity *17:* 27–61 (1962).

Durrant, A.: Induction and growth of flax genotrophs. Heredity *27:* 277–298 (1971).

Eagle, H.: The minimum vitamin requirements of the L and HeLa cells in tissue culture, the production of specific vitamin deficiencies and their cure. J. exp. Med. *102:* 595–600 (1955).

Eaves, G.: A consequence of normal diploid cell mortality. Mech. Age. Dev. *2:* 19–21 (1973).

Ebeling, A.H.: The permanent life of connective tissue outside of the organism. J. exp. Med. *17:* 273–285 (1913).

Edmunds, G.F.: May fly. Encycl. Br. *15:* 11 (1965).

Edney, E.B. and Gill, R.W.: Evolution of senescence and specific longevity. Nature, Lond. *220:* 281–282 (1968).

Eklund, J. and Bradford, G.E.: Longevity and lifetime body weight in mice selected for rapid growth. Nature, Lond. *265:* 48–49 (1977).

Elens, A.A.; Mouravieff, A.N., and Heuts, M.J.: The age of reproduction as a factor of transmissible divergences in learning ability in the mouse. Experientia *22:* 186–188 (1966).

Englert, D.C. and Bell, A.E.: Selection for time of pupation in *Tribolium castaneum.* Genetics *64:* 541–552 (1970).

Epstein, J.; Williams, J.R., and Little, J.B.: Deficient DNA repair in human progeroid cells. Proc. natn. Acad. Sci. USA *70:* 977–981 (1973).

Epstein, J.; Williams, J.R., and Little, J.B.: Rate of DNA repair in progeric and normal human fibroblasts. Biochem. biophys. Res. Commun. *59:* 850–857 (1974).

Failla, G.: The aging process and carcinogenesis. Ann. N.Y. Acad. Sci. *71:* 1124–1135 (1958).

Falconer, D.S.: Introduction to quantitative genetics (Oliver & Boyd, Edinburgh 1960).

Fallon, J.F. and Saunders, J.W.: In vitro analysis of the control of cell death in a zone of prospective necrosis from the chick wing bud. Devl Biol. *18:* 553–570 (1968).

Ferris, J.C.: Comparison of the life histories of mictic and amictic females in the rotifer, *Hydatina senta.* Biol. Bull. Wood's Hole *63:* 442 (1932).

Finch, C.E.: Enzyme activities, gene function and ageing in mammals. Review. Expl Gerontol. *7:* 53–67 (1972).

Fisher, R.A.: A preliminary linkage test with agouti and undulated mice. Heredity *3:* 229–241 (1949).

Flower, S.S.: Further notes on the duration of life in animals. III. Reptiles. Cairo Sci. J. *25:* 1 (1937).

Flower, S.S.: Further notes on the duration of life of animals. IV. Birds. Proc. zool. Soc. Lond. A 195 (1938).

Franke, W.W.; Berger, S.; Falk, H.; Spring, H.; Scheer, U.; Herth, W.; Trendelenburg, M.F., and Schweiger, H.G.: Morphology of the nucleo-cytoplasmic interactions during the development of *Acetabularia* cells. I. The vegetative phase. Protoplasma *82:* 249–282 (1974).

Frohawk, F.W.: Feeding butterflies in captivity. Entomologist *68:* 184 (1935).

Fulder, S.J.: Spontaneous mutations in ageing human cells: studies using a Herpesvirus probe. Mech. Age. Dev. *6:* 271–282 (1977).

Gajdusek, D.C. and Zigas, V.: Degenerative disease of the central nervous system in New Guinea. The endemic occurrence of 'Kuru' in the native population. New Engl. J. Med. *257:* 974–978 (1957).

Gates, W.H.: The Japanese waltzing mouse. Publ. Carneg. Inst. *337:* 83 (1926).

Gehring, W.J.: Developmental genetics of *Drosophila.* Annu. Rev. Genet. *10:* 209–252 (1976).

Gehring, W.J. and Nöthiger, R.: The imaginal discs of *Drosophila;* in *Counce and Waddington* Developmental systems. Insects, vol. 2, pp. 211–290 (Academic Press, London 1973).

Gershon, D. and Gershon, H.: An evaluation of the 'error catastrophe' theory of ageing in the light of recent experimental results. Gerontology *22:* 212–219 (1976).

Gershon, H. and Gershon, D.: Detection of inactive enzyme molecule in ageing organisms. Nature, Lond. *227:* 1214–1217 (1970).

Gershon, H. and Gershon, D.: Inactive enzyme molecules in aging mice: liver aldolase. Proc. natn. Acad. Sci. USA *70:* 909–913 (1973a).

Gershon, H. and Gershon, D.: Altered enzyme molecules in senescent organisms: mouse muscle aldolase. Mech. Age. Dev. *2:* 33–40 (1973b).

Gershon, H.; Zeelon, P., and Gershon, D.: Faulty proteins: altered gene products in senescent cells and organisms; in *Kohn and Shatkay* Control of gene expression, pp. 255–264 (Plenum Publishing, New York 1974).

Girardi, A.J.; Jensen, F.C., and Koprowski, H.: SV40-induced transformation of human diploid cells: crisis and recovery. J. cell. comp. Physiol. *65:* 69–78 (1965).

Glass, B.: Genes and the man (Bureau of Publications, Teachers College, Columbia University, New York 1943).

Glass, B.: Genetics of aging; in *Shock* Aging: some social and biological aspects, pp. 67–99 (Am. Association for the Advancement of Science, Washington 1960).

Glücksmann, A.: Cell deaths in normal vertebrate ontogeny. Biol. Rev. Cambridge phil. Soc. *26:* 59–86 (1951).

Goldberg, A.L.: Degradation of abnormal proteins in *Escherichia coli.* Proc. natn. Acad. Sci. USA *69:* 422–426 (1972).

Goldstein, S.: Life-span of cultured cells in progeria. Lancet *i:* 424 (1969).

Goldstein, S.; Littlefield, J.W., and Soeldner, J.S.: Diabetes mellitus and aging: diminished plating efficiency of cultured human fibroblasts. Proc. natn. Acad. Sci. USA *64:* 155–169 (1969).

Goldstein, S. and Moerman, E.J.: Defective proteins in normal and abnormal human fibroblasts during aging *in vitro.* Interdiscipl. Topics Gerontol., vol. 10, pp. 24–43 (Karger, Basel 1976).

Gonzalez, B.M.: Experimental studies on the duration of life. VIII. The influence upon duration of life of certain mutant genes of *Drosophila melanogaster.* Am. Nat. *57:* 289–325 (1923).

Gowen, J.W.: Genetic patterns in senescence and infection. J. Am. geriat. Soc. *10:* 107–124 (1962).

Grasse, P.P.: L'évolution du vivant (Albin Michel, Paris 1973).

Gray, J.: The growth of fish. III. The effect of temperature on the development of the eggs of *Salmo fario.* Br. J. exp. Biol. *6:* 125–130 (1929).

Graziosi, G. and Roberts, D.B.: Molecular anisotropy of the early *Drosophila* embryo. Nature, Lond. *258:* 157–159 (1975).

Grüneberg, H.: The genetics of the mouse (University Press, Cambridge 1943).

Grüneberg, H.: Hereditary lesions of the labyrinth in the mouse. Br. med. J. *i:* 153–157 (1956).

Gruwez, G.; Hoste, C.; Lints, C.V., and Lints, F.A.: Oviposition rhythm in *Drosophila melanogaster* and its alteration by a change in the photoperiodicity. Experientia *27:* 1414–1416 (1971).

Gurdon, J.B.: The control of gene expression in animal development (Clarendon Press, Oxford 1976).

Gurdon, J.B. and Brown, D.D.: Cytoplasmic regulation of RNA synthesis and nucleolus formation in developing embryos of *Xenopus laevis.* J. molec. Biol. *12:* 27–35 (1965).

Gurdon, J.B. and Woodland, H.R.: The cytoplasmic control of nuclear activity in animal development. Biol. Rev. *43:* 233–267 (1968).

Guthrie, R.D.: Senescence as an adaptive trait. Perspect. Biol. Med. *12:* 313–324 (1969).

Haemmerling, J.: Nucleo-cytoplasmic interactions in *Acetabularia* and other cells. Annu. Rev. Plant Physiol. *14:* 65–92 (1963).

Hahn, H.P. von: Control of cellular ageing at the genome: the regulation of transcription. Proc. 8th Int. Congr. Gerontol., 1969, vol. 1, pp. 134–137.

Hahn, H.P. von: Failures of regulation mechanisms as causes of cellular aging. Adv. Gerontol. Res. *3:* 1–38 (1971).

Hahn, H.P. von: Primary causes of ageing: a brief review of some modern theories and concepts. Mech. Age. Dev. *2:* 245–250 (1973).

Hansson, A.A.: A tissue culture study of inherited dystrophy of the retina in mice. Arch. Pathol. Anat. Physiol. *340:* 69–83 (1965).

Harris, H.; Miller, O.J.; Klein, G.; Worst, P., and Tachibana, T.: Suppression of malignancy by cell fusion. Nature, Lond. *223:* 363–368 (1969).

Harrison, B.J. and Holliday, R.: Senescence and the fidelity of protein synthesis in *Drosophila.* Nature, Lond. *213:* 990–992 (1967).

Harrison, P.R.; Hell, A.; Birnie, G.D., and Paul, J.: Evidence for single copies of globin genes in the mouse genome. Nature, Lond. *239:* 219–221 (1972).

Hart, R.W. and Setlow, R.B.: Correlation between deoxyribonucleic acid excision-repair and life-span in a number of mammalian species. Proc. natn. Acad. Sci. USA *71:* 2169–2173 (1974).

Hart, R.W. and Setlow, R.B.: DNA repair in late-passage human cells. Mech. Age. Dev. *5:* 67–77 (1976).

Hay, R.J. and Strehler, B.L.: The limited growth span of cell strains isolated from the chick embryo. Expl Gerontol. *2:* 123–135 (1967).

Hayflick, L.: The limited *in vitro* lifetime of human diploid cell strains. Expl Cell Res. *37:* 614–637 (1965).

Hayflick, L.: The biology of human aging. Am. J. med. Sci. *265:* 432–445 (1973).

Hayflick, L. and Moorhead, P.S.: The serial cultivation of human diploid cell strains. Expl Cell Res. *25:* 585–621 (1961).

Henshaw, P.S.; Riley, E.R., and Stapleton, G.E.: The biological effects of pile radiations. Radiology *49:* 349–364 (1947).

Herrick, F.H.: Natural history of the American lobster. Bull. US Bureau Fish. *29:* 149 (1911).

Heuts, M.J.: Nieuwe problematiek in de genetica. Agricultura *4:* 342–352 (1956).

Hitotsumachi, S.; Rabinowitz, Z., and Sachs, L.: Chromosomal control of reversion in transformed cells. Nature, Lond. *231:* 511–514 (1971).

Holland, J.J.; Kohne, D., and Doyle, M.V.: Analysis of virus replication in ageing human fibroblast cultures. Nature, Lond. *245:* 316–319 (1973).

Holliday, R.: Testing the protein error theory of ageing: a reply to Baird, Samis, Massie and Zimmerman. Gerontologia *21:* 64–68 (1975).

Holliday, R.; Porterfield, J.S., and Gibbs, D.D.: Premature ageing and occurrence of altered enzyme in Werner's syndrome fibroblasts. Nature, Lond. *248:* 762–763 (1974).

Holliday, R. and Tarrant, G.M.: Altered enzymes in ageing human fibroblasts. Nature, Lond. *238:* 26–30 (1972).

Holt, S.B.: The genetics of dermal ridges (Thomas, Springfield 1968).

Horn, S.N. van: Studies on the embryogenesis of *Aulocara elliotti* (Thomas) (Orthoptera, Acrididae). II. Developmental variability and the effects of maternal age and environment. J. Morph. *120:* 115–134 (1966).

Hoste, C.: Influence de l'âge parental dans des expériences de sélection chez *Drosophila melanogaster;* thèse de doctorat, Louvain (1975).

Hotta, Y. and Benzer, S.: Mapping of behaviour in *Drosophila* mosaics. Nature, Lond. *240:* 527–535 (1972).

Hyde, R.R.: Inheritance of the length of life in *Drosophila ampelophila.* Indiana Acad. Sci. Rep. *1913:* 113–123.

Illmensee, K. and Mintz, B.: Totipotency and normal differentiation of single teratocarcinoma cells cloned by injection into blastocysts. Proc. natn. Acad. Sci. USA *73:* 549–553 (1976).

Jacobson, M.F.; Asso, J., and Baltimore, D.: Further evidence on the formation of poliovirus proteins. J. molec. Biol. *49:* 657–669 (1970).

Jalavisto, E.: Inheritance of longevity according to Finnish and Swedish genealogies. Annls Med. intern. Fenn. *40:* 263–274 (1951).

Jennings, H.S. and Lynch, R.S.: Age, mortality, fertility, and individual diversities in the rotifer *Proales sordida* Gosse. I. Effects of age of the parent on characteristics of the offspring. J. exp. Zool. *50:* 345–407 (1928).

Jensen, A.R.: Estimation of the limits of heritability of traits by comparison of mono- and dizygotic twins. Proc. natn. Acad. Sci. USA *58:* 149–156 (1967).

Jinks, J.L.: Somatic selection in fungi. Nature, Lond. *174:* 409–410 (1954).

Jinks, J.L.: Naturally occurring cytoplasmic changes in fungi. C.r. Lab. Carlsberg *26:* 183–203 (1956).

Johnson, F. and Strong, L.C.: The effect of maternal age on time of first litters in inbred mice. J. Geront. *18:* 246–249 (1963).

Kallmann, F.J.: Twin data on the genetics of ageing; in *Wolstenholme and O'Connor* Methodology of the study of ageing. Ciba Found. Coll. on Ageing, 1957, vol. 3, pp. 131–148.

Kallmann, F.J.; Aschner, B.M., and Falek, A.: Comparative data on longevity, adjustment to aging, and causes of death in a senescent twin population. Novant'anni delle Leggi Mendeliane, pp. 330–339 (1956).

Kallmann, F.J. and Sander, G.: Twin studies on aging and longevity. J. Hered. *39:* 349–357 (1948).

Kalthoff, K.: Position of targets and period of competence for UV-induction of the malformation 'double abdomen' in the egg of *Smittia* spec. (Diptera. Chironomidae). Roux Arch. EntwMech. Org. *168:* 63–84 (1971).

Kandler-Singer, I. and Kalthoff, K.: RNase sensitivity of an anterior morphogenetic determinant in an insect egg (*Smittia* sp., Chironomidae, Diptera). Proc. natn. Acad. Sci. USA *73:* 3739–3743 (1976).

Kedes, L.H. and Birnstiel, M.L.: Reiteration and clustering of DNA sequences complementary to histone messenger RNA. Nature new Biol. *230:* 165–169 (1971).

Kobozieff, N.: Mortalité et âge limite chez la souris. C.r. Séanc. Soc. Biol. *106:* 704 (1931).

Krause, G. and Sander, K.: Ooplasmic reaction systems in insect oogenesis. Adv. Morphol. *2:* 259–303 (1962).

Labitte, A.: Longévité de quelques insectes en captivité. Bull. Mus. Hist. nat. Paris *22:* 105 (1916).

Lansing, A.I.: A transmissible, cumulative and reversible factor in aging. J. Geront. *2:* 228–239 (1947).

Lansing, A.I.: Evidence for aging as a consequence of growth cessation. Proc. natn. Acad. Sci. USA *34:* 304–310 (1948).

Lansing, A.I.: A nongenic factor in the longevity of rotifers. Ann. N.Y. Acad. Sci. *57:* 455–464 (1954).

Lansing, A.I.: Comparative physiology of aging. Fed. Proc. Fed. Am. Socs exp. Biol. *15:* 960–964 (1956).

Lawrence, P.A.: The organization of the insect segment. Symp. Soc. exp. Biol. *25:* 379–391 (1971).

Lawrence, P.A.: RNA and generation of positional information. Nature, Lond. *264:* 604 (1976).

Lawrence, P.A.; Crick, F.H.C., and Munro, M.: A gradient of positional information in an insect, *Rhodnius.* J. Cell Sci. *11:* 815–853 (1972).

Lerner, I.M.: Genetic homeostasis (Oliver & Boyd, Edinburgh 1954).

Lesher, S.; Fry, R.J.M., and Kohn, H.I.: Influence of age on transit time of cells of mouse intestinal epithelium. Lab. Invest. *10:* 291–300 (1961).

Lewis, C.M. and Holliday, R.: Mistranslation and ageing in *Neurospora.* Nature, Lond. *228:* 877–880 (1970).

Linn, S.; Kairis, M., and Holliday, R.: Decreased fidelity of DNA polymerase in aging human fibroblasts. Proc. natn. Acad. Sci. USA *73:* 2818–2822 (1976).

Lints, C.V.; Lints, F.A., and Zeuthen, E.: Respiration in *Drosophila.* I. Oxygen consumption during development of the egg in genotypes of *Drosophila melanogaster* with contribution to the gradient diver technique. C.r. Trav. Lab. Carlsberg *36:* 35–66 (1967).

Lints, F.A.: Size in relation to development time and egg-density in *Drosophila melanogaster.* Nature, Lond. *197:* 1128–1130 (1963).

Lints, F.A.: Life-span in *Drosophila.* Gerontologia *17:* 33–51 (1971).

Lints, F.A. and Beardmore, J.: Variation of heritability as a function of parental age in *Drosophila melanogaster.* Proc. 10th Int. Congr. Gerontol., vol. 2, p. 22 (1975).

Lints, F.A. and Gruwez, G.: What determines the duration of development in *Drosophila melanogaster?* Mech. Age. Dev. *1:* 285–297 (1972).

Lints, F.A. and Hoste, C.: The Lansing effect revisited. I. Life-span. Expl Gerontol. *9:* 51–69 (1974).

Lints, F.A. and Hoste, C.: The Lansing effect revisited. II. Cumulative and spontaneously reversible parental age effects on fecundity in *Drosophila melanogaster.* Evolution *31:* 387–404 (1977).

Lints, F.A. and Lints, C.V.: Influence of preimaginal environment on fecundity and ageing in *Drosophila melanogaster* hybrids. I. Preimaginal population density. Expl Gerontol. *4:* 231–244 (1969).

Lints, F.A. and Lints, C.V.: Relationship between growth and ageing in *Drosophila.* Nature, Lond. *229:* 86–87 (1971a).

Lints, F.A. and Lints, C.V.: Influence of preimaginal environment on fecundity and ageing in *Drosophila melanogaster* hybrids. II. Preimaginal temperature. Expl Gerontol. *6:* 417–426 (1971b).

Lints, F.A. and Lints, C.V.: Influence of preimaginal environment on fecundity and ageing in *Drosophila melanogaster* hybrids. III. Developmental speed and life-span. Expl Gerontol. *6:* 427–445 (1971c).

Lints, F.A. and Parisi, P.: Heritability and parental age: a twin study on finger ridge count. 2nd Int. Congr. Twin Studies, 1977, No. 9.

Lints, F.A.; Parisi, P., and Gedda, L.: Parental age and the heritability of finger ridge count. 5th Int. Congr. Human Genetics, 1976.

Lints, F.A. and Soliman, M.H.: Growth rate and longevity in *Drosophila melanogaster* and *Tribolium castaneum.* Nature, Lond. *266:* 624–625 (1977).

Lints, F.A. and Stoll, J.: Selection for life-span in *Drosophila* (in preparation).

Løvtrup, S.: Epigenetics (Wiley & Sons, Chichester 1974).

Løvtrup, S.: La crise du darwinisme. Recherche *8:* 642–649 (1977).

Ludwig, D. and Fiore, C.: Further studies on the relationship between parental age and the life cycle of the mealworm, *Tenebrio molitor.* Annls entomol. Soc. Am. *53:* 595–600 (1960).

Ludwig, D. and Fiore, C.: Effects of parental age on offspring from isolated pairs of the mealworm *Tenebrio molitor.* Annls entomol. Soc. Am. *54:* 463–464 (1961).

Macieira-Coelho, A.: Action of cortisone on human fibroblasts *in vitro.* Experientia *22:* 390–391 (1966).

Macieira-Coelho, A.: Metabolism of ageing cells in culture: introduction. Gerontology *22:* 3–8 (1976).

Macieira-Coelho, A.; Diatloff, C., and Malaise, E.: Concept of fibroblast aging *in vitro:* implications for cell biology. Gerontology *23:* 290–305 (1977).

Macieira-Coelho, A. and Lima, L.: Aging *in vitro:* incorporation of RNA and protein precursors and acid phosphatase activity during the life span of chick embryo fibroblasts. Mech. Age. Dev. *2:* 13–18 (1973).

Martin, G.H.; Sprague, C.A., and Epstein, C.J.: Replicative life-span of cultivated human cells: effects of donor's age, tissue and genotype. Lab. Invest. *23:* 86–92 (1970).

Mather, K.: Crossing over. Biol. Rev. *13:* 252–292 (1938).

Mather, K. and Jinks, J.L.: Cytoplasm in sexual reproduction. Nature, Lond. *182:* 1188–1190 (1958).

Mather, K. and Jinks, J.L.: Biometrical genetics (Chapman & Hall, London 1971).

Maynard Smith, J.: The rate of ageing in *Drosophila subobscura;* in *Wolstenholme and O'Connor* The lifespan of animals. Ciba Found. Coll. on Ageing, 1959, vol. 5, pp. 269–285.

Maynard Smith, J.; Bozcuk, A.N., and Tebbutt, S.: Protein turnover in adult *Drosophila.* J. Insect Physiol. *16:* 601–613 (1970).

McCay, C.M.; Crowell, M.F., and Maynard, L.A.: The effect of retarded growth upon the length of the life span and upon the ultimate body size. J. Nutr. *10:* 63–79 (1935).

McCay, C.M.; Maynard, L.A.; Sperling, G., and Barnes, L.L.: Retarded growth, life span, ultimate body size and age changes in the albino rat after feeding diets restricted in calories. J. Nutr. *18:* 1–13 (1939).

McDonald, R.A.: Life span of liver cells. Archs intern. Med. *107:* 335–343 (1961).

McHale, J.S.; Mouton, M.L., and McHale, J.T.: Limited culture lifespan of human diploid cells as a function of metabolic time instead of division potential. Expl Gerontol. *6:* 89–93 (1971).

Medawar, P.B.: An unsolved problem of biology (Lewis, London 1952).

Medvedev, Z.A.: Repetition of molecular-genetic information as a possible factor in evolutionary changes of life span. Expl Gerontol. *7:* 227–238 (1972).

Medvedev, Z.A.: Aging and longevity. New approaches and new perspectives. Gerontologist *15:* 196–201 (1975).

Mellen, I.: The science and mystery of the cat (Scribner, New York 1940).

Mertz, D.B.: Senescent decline in flour beetle strains selected for early adult fitness. Physiol. Zool. *48:* 1–23 (1975).

Milkman, R.D.: Temperature effects on day old *Drosophila* pupae. J. gen. Physiol. *45:* 777–799 (1962).

Milkman, R.D.: Kinetic analysis of temperature adaptation in *Drosophila* pupae; in Molecular mechanisms of temperature adaptation, pp. 147–162 (Am. Association for the Advancement of Science, Washington 1967).

Milo, G.E.: Enhancement of senescence in low passage human embryonic lung cells by an agent extracted from phase III cells. Expl Cell Res. *79:* 143–151 (1973).

Mintz, B. and Illmensee, K.: Normal genetically mosaic mice produced from malignant teratocarcinoma cells. Proc. natn. Acad. Sci. USA *72:* 3585–3589 (1975).

Mitra, J.; Mapes, M.O., and Stewards, F.C.: Growth and organized development of cultured cells. IV. The behaviour of the nucleus. Am. J. Bot. *47:* 357–368 (1960).

Mohr, E.: Lebensdauer einiger Tiere in zoologischen Gärten. Zool. Gärt., Lpz. *18:* 60 (1951).

Mühlbock, O.: Factors influencing the life-span of inbred mice. Gerontologia *3:* 177–183 (1959).

Muller, H.J.: Mechanisms of life-span shortening; in *Harris* Cellular basis and aetiology of late somatic effects of ionizing radiation (Academic Press, New York 1963).

Murphy, J.S. and Davidoff, M.: The result of improved nutrition on the Lansing effect in *Moina macrocopa.* Biol. Bull. *142:* 302–309 (1972).

O'Brian, D.M.: Effects of parental age on the life cycle of *Drosophila melanogaster.* Annls entomol. Soc. Am. *54:* 412–416 (1961).

Orgel, L.E.: The maintenance of the accuracy of protein synthesis and its relevance to ageing. Proc. natn. Acad. Sci. USA *49:* 517–521 (1963).

Orgel, L.E.: Ageing of clones of mammalian cells. Nature, Lond. *243:* 441–445 (1973).

Osborne, T.B. and Mendel, L.B.: The resumption of growth after long continued failure to grow. J. biol. Chem. *23:* 439–455 (1915).

Osborne, T.B. and Mendel, L.B.: Acceleration of growth after retardation. Am. J. Physiol., Lond. *40:* 16–20 (1916).

Osborne, T.B.; Mendel, L.B., and Ferry, E.L.: The effect of retardation of growth upon the breeding period and duration of life of rats. Science, N.Y. *45:* 294–295 (1917).

Packer, L. and Fuehr, K.: Low oxygen concentration extends the lifespan of cultured diploid cells. Nature, Lond. *267:* 423–425 (1977).

Packer, L. and Smith, J.R.: Extension of the lifespan of cultured normal human diploid cells by vitamin E. Proc. natn. Acad. Sci. USA *71:* 4763–4767 (1974).

Parsons, P.A.: Maternal age and developmental variability. J. exp. Biol. *39:* 251–260 (1962).

Parsons, P.A.: Parental age and the offspring. Q. Rev. Biol. *39:* 258–275 (1964).

Pearl, R.: Introduction to medical biometry and statistics; 3rd ed. (Saunders, Philadelphia 1940).

Pearl, R. and Parker, S.L.: Experimental studies on the duration of life. II. Hereditary differences in duration of life in line-bred strains of *Drosophila.* Am. Nat. *56:* 174–187 (1922a).

Pearl, R. and Parker, S.L.: Experimental studies on the duration of life. V. On the influence of certain environmental factors on duration of life in *Drosophila.* Am. Nat. *56:* 385–398 (1922b).

Pellie, C.; Briard, M.L.; Feingold, J., and Frezal, J.: Parental age in retinoblastoma. Humangenetik *20:* 59–62 (1973).

Pendergrass, W.R.; Martin, G.M., and Bornstein, P.: Evidence contrary to the protein error hypothesis for *in vitro* senescence. J. cell. Physiol. *87:* 3–14 (1975).

Penrose, L.S. and Smith, G.F.: Down's anomaly (Little, Brown, Boston 1966).

Pierce, G.B.: Differentiation of normal and malignant cells. Fed. Proc. Fed. Am. Socs exp. Biol. *29:* 1248–1254 (1970).

Pierce, G.B. and Johnson, L.D.: Differentiation and cancer. In vitro *7:* 140–145 (1971).

Pitha, J.; Adams, R., and Pitha, P.M.: Viral probe into the events of cellular *(in vitro)* aging. J. cell. Physiol. *83:* 211–218 (1974).

Pitha, J.; Stork, E., and Wimmer, E.: Protein synthesis during aging of human cells in culture. Direction by polio virus. Expl Cell Res. *94:* 310–314 (1975).

Ponten, J.: The growth capacity of normal and Rous virus transformed chicken fibroblasts *in vitro.* Int. J. Cancer *6:* 323–332 (1970).

Ponten, J.: Spontaneous and virus induced transformation in cell culture. Virol. Monogr. No. 8, p. 25 (Springer, Berlin 1971).

Quincey, R. and Wilson, S.: The utilization of genes for ribosomal RNA, 5 sRNA and transfer RNA in liver cells of adult rats. Proc. natn. Acad. Sci. USA *64:* 981 (1969).

Rabinowitz, Z. and Sachs, L.: The formation of variants with a reversion of properties of transformed cells. V. Reversion to a limited life-span. Int. J. Cancer *6:* 388–398 (1970a).

Rabinowitz, Z. and Sachs, L.: Control of the reversion of properties in transformed cells. Nature, Lond. *225:* 136–139 (1970b).

Rabinowitz, Z. and Sachs, L.: The formation of variants with a reversion of properties of transformed cells. VIII. *In vitro* limited life span of variants isolated from tumors. Int. J. Cancer *10:* 607–612 (1972).

Regan, J.D. and Setlow, R.B.: DNA repair in human progeroid cells. Biochem. biophys. Res. Commun. *59:* 858–864 (1974).

Reincke, V.; Burlington, H.; Cronkite, E.P., and Laissve, J.: Hayflick's hypothesis: an approach to *in vivo* testing; in *Thorbecke* Biology of aging and development (Plenum Publishing, New York 1975).

Reiss, U. and Rothstein, M.: Heat-labile isozymes of isocitrate lyase from aging *Turbatrix aceti.* Biochem. biophys. Res. Commun. *61:* 1012–1016 (1974).

Reiss, U. and Rothstein, M.: Age-related changes in isocitrate lyase from the free-living nematode, *Turbatrix aceti.* J. biol. Chem. *250:* 826–830 (1975).

Richards, A.G. and Kolderie, M.Q.: Variation in weight, developmental rate, and hatchability of *Oncopeltus* eggs as a function of the mother's age. Entomol. News *68:* 57–64 (1957).

Roberts, D.F. and Bear, J.: Genetics and ageing in man (in preparation).

Roberts, R.C.: The lifetime growth and reproduction of selected strains of mice. Heredity *16:* 369–381 (1961).

Rockstein, M.: Heredity and longevity in the animal kingdom. J. Geront. *13:* suppl. 2, pp. 7–12 (1958).

Rockstein, M. (ed.): Theoretical aspects of aging (Academic Press, New York 1974a).

Rockstein, M.: The genetic basis for longevity; in *Rockstein* Theoretical aspects of aging, pp. 1–10 (Academic Press, New York 1974b).

Ross, M.H.: Protein, calories and life expectancy. Fed. Proc. Fed. Am. Socs exp. Biol. *18:* 1190–1207 (1959).

Ross, M.H.; Lustbader, E., and Bras, G.: Dietary practices and growth responses as predictors of longevity. Nature, Lond. *262:* 548–553 (1976).

Rothfels, K.H.; Kupelwieser, E.B., and Parker, R.C.: Effects of X-irradiated feeder layers on mitotic activity and development of aneuploidy in mouse embryo cells *in vitro.* Proc. Can. Cancer Conf. *5:* 191–223 (1963).

Ryan, J.M.; Duda, G., and Cristofalo, V.J.: Error accumulation and aging in human diploid cells. J. Geront. *29:* 616–621 (1974).

Sacher, G.A.: Molecular versus systemic theories on the genesis of ageing. Expl Gerontol. *3:* 265–271 (1968).

Saunders, J.W., jr. and Fallon, J.F.: Cell death in morphogenesis; in *Locke* Current status of some major problems in developmental biology. 25th Symp. Soc. Dev. Biol., pp. 289–314 (Academic Press, New York 1967).

Saunders, J.W., jr.; Gasseling, M.T., and Saunders, L.C.: Cellular death in morphogenesis of the avian wing. Devl Biol. *5:* 147–178 (1962).

Schaechter, M.; Maaløe, O., and Kjeldgaard, N.O.: Dependency on medium and temperature of cell size and chemical composition during balanced growth of *Salmonella typhimurium.* J. gen. Microbiol. *19:* 592–606 (1958).

Schneider, E.L. and Chase, G.A.: Relationship between age of donor and *in vitro* life span of human diploid fibroblasts. Interdiscipl. Topics Geront., vol. 10, pp. 62–69 (Karger, Basel 1976).

Scott, E.J. van and Ekel, T.M.: Kinetics of hyperplasia in psoriasis. Archs Derm. *88:* 373–381 (1963).

Searle, A.G.: The influence of maternal age on development of the skeleton of the mouse. Ann. N.Y. Acad. Sci. *57:* 558–563 (1954).

Setlow, R.B.; Regan, J.D.; German, J., and Carrier, W.L.: Evidence that xeroderma pigmentosum cells do not perform the first step in the repair of ultraviolet damage to their DNA. Proc. natn. Acad. Sci. USA *64:* 1035–1041 (1969).

Shami, S.A.: Stabilizing selection, heterozygosity and parental age effects in the guppy *Poecilia reticulata* (Peters) and *Drosophila melanogaster;* PhD thesis, Swansea (1977).

Sheldrake, A.R.: The ageing, growth and death of cells. Nature, Lond. *250:* 381–385 (1974).

Sheng, T.C.: The genetic basis of woolly degeneration in *Neurospora crassa.* Bot. Gaz. *113:* 203–206 (1951).

Silberberg, M. and Silberberg, R.: Diet and life span. Physiol. Rev. *35:* 347–362 (1955).

Smith-Sonneborn, J.; Klass, M., and Cotton, D.: Parental age and life span versus progeny life span in *Paramecium.* J. Cell Sci. *14:* 691–699 (1974).

Snow, M.H.C.: Maternal effects on development. Nature, Lond. *260:* 94 (1976).

Sober, H.A.: Handbook of biochemistry, pp. H112–H114 (Chem. Rubber Co., Cleveland 1970).

Sokal, R.R.: Senescence and genetic load: evidence from *Tribolium.* Science, N.Y. *167:* 1733–1734 (1970).

Soliman, M.H. and Lints, F.A.: Longevity, growth rate and related traits among strains of *Tribolium castaneum.* Gerontologia *21:* 102–116 (1975).

Soliman, M.H. and Lints, F.A.: Bibliography on longevity, ageing and parental age effects in *Drosophila.* Gerontology *22:* 380–410 (1976).

Sonneborn, T.M.: Genetic studies on *Stenostomum incaudatum* (Nov. Spec.). I. The nature and origin of differences among individuals formed during vegetative reproduction. J. exp. Zool. *57:* 57–108 (1930).

Sonneborn, T.M.: Does preformed cell structure play an essential role in cell heredity? in *Allen* The nature of biological diversity, pp. 165–221 (McGraw-Hill, New York (1963).

Sonneborn, T.M.: Gene action in development. Proc. R. Soc. B *176:* 347–366 (1970).

Sonneborn, T.M.: Paramecium aurelia; in *King* Handbook of genetics, vol. 2, pp. 469–593 (Plenum Publishing, New York 1974).

Sorsby, A.P.; Koller, C.; Attfield, M.; Davey, J.B., and Lucas, D.R.: Retinal dystrophy in the mouse: histological and genetic aspects. J. exp. Zool. *125:* 171–198 (1954).

Spaas, J.T. and Heuts, M.J.: Contributions to the comparative physiology and genetics of the European Salmonidae. II. Physiologie et génétique du développement embryonnaire. Hydrobiologia *12:* 1–26 (1958).

Stanley, J.F.; Pye, D., and MacGregor, A.: Comparison of doubling numbers attained by cultured animal cells with life span of species. Nature, Lond. *255:* 158–159 (1975).

Stephenson, R.A.: British sea anemones (The Ray Society, London 1935).

Stevenson, K.G. and Curtis, H.J.: Chromosomal aberrations in irradiated and nitrogen mustard treated mice. Radiat. Res. *15:* 744–784 (1961).

Steward, F.C.: Growth and organization in plants (Addison-Wesley, Reading 1968).

Steward, F.C.; Mapes, M.D., and Smith, J.: Growth and organized development of cultured cells. I. Growth and division of freely suspended cells. Am. J. Bot. *45:* 693–703 (1958a).

Steward, F.C.; Mapes, M.O., and Mears, K.: Growth and organized development of cultured cells. II. Organization in cultures grown from freely suspended cells. Am. J. Bot. *45:* 705–708 (1958b).

Steward, F.C.; Shantz, E.M.; Pollard, J.K.; Mapes, M.O., and Mitra, J.: Growth induction in explanted cells and tissues: metabolic and morphogenetic manifestations; in *Rudnick* Synthesis of molecular and cellular structure (Ronald Press, New York 1961).

Stoll, J.: Etude du déterminisme de la longévité chez *Drosophila melanogaster;* Mémoire de fin d'études, Louvain (1977).

Strehler, B.L.: Cellular aging. Ann. N.Y. Acad. Sci. *138:* 661–679 (1967).

Strong, L.C.: Production of the CBA strain of inbred mice: long life associated with low tumour incidence. Br. J. exp. Path. *17:* 60-63 (1936).

Strong, L.C. (ed.): Parental age and the characteristics of the offspring. Symp. N.Y. Acad. Sci. (1954).

Strong, L.C.: Biological aspects of cancer and aging (Pergamon Press, Oxford 1968).

Sussman, M.: Model for quantitative and qualitative control of mRNA translation in eukaryotes. Nature, Lond. *225:* 1245–1246 (1970).

Swim, H.E. and Parker, R.F.: Culture characteristics of human fibroblasts propagated serially. Am. J. Hyg. *66:* 235–243 (1957).

Szilard, L.: On the nature of the aging process. Proc. natn. Acad. Sci. USA *45:* 30–45 (1959).

Terra, N. de: Evidence for cell surface control of macronuclear DNA synthesis in *Stentor.* Nature, Lond. *258:* 300–303 (1975).

Tice, R.R. and Schneider, E.L.: In vitro aspects of human genetic disorders which feature accelerated aging. Interdiscipl. Topics Geront., vol. 9, pp. 60–68 (Karger, Basel 1976).

Todaro, G.J. and Green, H.: Quantitative studies of the growth of mouse embryo cells in culture and their development into established lines. J. Cell Biol. *17:* 299–313 (1963).

Tomkins, G.A.; Stanbridge, E.J., and Hayflick, L.: Viral probes of aging in the human diploid cell strain Wl –38 (38110). Proc. Soc. exp. Biol. Med. *146:* 385–390 (1974).

Torrey, J.G.: Morphogenesis in relation to chromosomal constitution in long-term tissue cultures. Physiol. Plant. *20:* 266–275 (1967).

Tracey, K.M.: Effects of parental age on the life cycle of the mealworm, *Tenebrio molitor* Linnaeus. Ann. entomol. Soc. Am. *51:* 429–432 (1958).

Tsien, H.C. and Wattiaux, J.M.: Effect of maternal age on DNA and RNA content of *Drosophila* eggs. Nature new Biol. *230:* 147–148 (1971).

Tünte, W.; Becker, P.E. und Knorre, G. von: Zur Genetic der Myositis ossificans progressiva. Humangenetik *4:* 320 (1967).

Valentin, J.: Selection for altered recombination frequency in *Drosophila melanogaster.* Hereditas *74:* 295–297 (1973).

Vogel, F. and Rathenberg, R.: Spontaneous mutation in man; in *Harris and Hirschorn* Adv. hum. Genet. *5:* 223–318 (1975).

Wallace, B.: Genetics and the great IQ controversy. Am. biol. Teacher *37:* 12–19 (1975).

Wattiaux, J.M.: Variation of bristle number in relation to speed of development in *Drosophila melanogaster.* Nature, Lond. *194:* 706–707 (1962).

Wattiaux, J.M.: Parental age effects in *Drosophila pseudoobscura.* Expl Gerontol. *3:* 55–61 (1968a).

Wattiaux, J.M.: Cumulative parental age effects in *Drosophila subobscura.* Evolution *22:* 406–421 (1968b).

Wattiaux, J.M. and Heuts, M.J.: Cyclic variation of bristle number with parental age in *Drosophila melanogaster.* Proc. 11th Int. Congr. Genetics, 1963, vol. 1, p. 168.

Wiener, F.; Klein, G., and Harris, H.: The analysis of malignancy by cell fusion. J. Cell Sci. *16:* 189–198 (1974).

Williams, G.C.: Pleiotropy, natural selection, and the evolution of senescence. Evolution *11:* 398–411 (1957).

Williamson, A.R. and Askonas, B.A.: Senescence of an antibody-forming cell clone. Nature, Lond. *238:* 337–339 (1972).

Wilson, E.B.: On cleavage and mosaic work; in *Crumpton* Experimental studies on gastropod development. Roux Arch. EntwMech. Org., Appendix *8:* 19 (1896).

Wilson, P.D.: Enzyme changes in ageing mammals. Gerontologia *19:* 79–125 (1973).

Wolpert, L.: Positional information and the spatial pattern of cellular differentiation. J. theor. Biol. *25:* 1–47 (1969).

Wolpert, L. and Lewis, J.H.: Towards a theory of development. Fed. Proc. Fed. Am. Socs exp. Biol. *34:* 14–20 (1975).

Woolhouse, H.W.: Longevity and senescence in plants. Sci. Progr. Oxford *61:* 123–147 (1974).

Wright, S.: Effects of age of parents on characteristics of the offspring. Am. Nat. *60:* 552–559 (1926).

Wright, S.: The genetics of vital characters of the guinea pig. Symp. Mammal. Genetics and Reproduction, 1960, pp. 123–151.

Yamamoto, T.; Rabinowitz, Z., and Sachs, L.: Identification of the chromosomes that control malignancy. Nature new Biol. *243:* 247–250 (1973).

Zeelon, P.; Gershon, H., and Gershon, D.: Inactive enzyme molecules in aging organisms. Nematode fructose-1,6-diphosphate aldolase. Biochemistry, N.Y. *12:* 1743–1750 (1973).

Zwilling, E.: Controlled degeneration during development; in *Reuck and Cameron* Cellular injury, pp. 352–362 (Churchill, London 1964).

Author Index

Subject Index

-, stem 54, 56
- strain culture 26−30, 100
- - -, IMR-90 29
- - -, MRC-5 31, 34
- - -, WI-38 22, 29, 33, 39, 58
- tumour 42, 44
-, vegetal 41
Cercus pedunculatus 5
Chicken embryo development 55, 57
- fibroblasts 40
- life-span 29
Chlamydomonas reinhardii 92
Chromosome aberrations 19−22, 41−43
-, transformation and 39
- unbalance 43
Colomba livia 5
Collagen 26
Competence 54−56
Complementation analysis 39
Conidia 75, 76
Conjugation 67, 92
Correlated response 47
Correlation coefficient 9, 10, 16, 22, 27
Cortisone 28
Crossbreeding 11−14
Cytoplasmic alternative steady states 98
- composition 53, 54, 61, 91
see also Molecular geography
- control 78
- organization 91
- rejuvenation 75−77

Daucus carotta, see Carrot
Death clock 55, 57
Dedifferentiation 44
see also Differentiation
Deprogrammation 43
see also Programme
Development 18, 19, 23, 91
see also Differentiation; Growth
-, parental age and 65
-, programmed 1, 18, 55
Developmental heterochrony 55
Diet 45, 46, 48−50, 99
see also Life-span, dietary habits
Differentiation 18, 19, 49
see also Development; Growth
-, cell death and 54, 56
-, control of 78, 91
- of tumour cells 44

Disease 10, 18, 20, 24, 49
DNA 25
- content in *Drosophila* eggs 66, 89, 90, 94
- - in flax 72
- - in mammalian cells 21
-, excision repair 22, 24, 31
- polymerase 31
-, single-strand breaks 22
- synthesis 91
- -, scheduled 22
- -, unscheduled 21, 22
Dog 4, 18, 20, 21
Double-abdomen 90
Down's syndrome 30, 62, 63
Drosophila 5, 9
- *melanogaster,* amino acid analogues and 25, 26, 34−36
- - bristles 66, 67, 88, 95
- -, DNA in eggs of 66, 89, 90, 94
- -, duration of development 51, 52, 66, 94, 95, 97
- - egg cytoplasm 90
- - egg size 66, 94
- - growth rate 51−53
- - heritability 69, 70, 72
- - hybrid 13, 35
- - imaginal discs 101
- -, inbred 12, 13
- -, Lansing effects in 82, 87−89, 97
- - larvae 26, 34
- - life-span 10−12, 35, 36, 51, 52, 87, 88, 95
- - mosaics 90
- - mutants 11
- -, non-disjunction in 64
- -, oxygen consumption 95
- -, preimaginal stages 51
- - pupae 96
- -, recombination frequency in 61−63, 66, 71
- -, RNA in eggs of 66, 89, 90, 94
- -, selection in 52
- - wing size 66−68
- *persimilis* 73
- *prosaltans* 73
- *pseudoobscura* 82
- *subobscura* and amino acid analogues 35
- - hybrids 13, 14, 16, 17
- - inbreds 13, 14, 16, 17

Drosophila subobscura (continued)
– –, Lansing effects in 82
– – life-span 13, 14, 16, 17
– *virilis* 54
Duck 23

E (expression) factors 39
Elephant 5, 21
Embryogenesis 54, 79, 89, 95
Enzymes 24, 25, 31
–, DNA polymerase 31
–, fructose 1,6-diphosphate aldolase 38
–, glucose-6-phosphate dehydrogenase 30, 31
–, glutamine dehydrogenase 31
–, isocitrate lyase 38
–, leucyl-t-RNA-synthetase 31
–, RNase 90
Ephemera, see Mayfly
Epidermis 53
Epiphanes brachionus 5
Equus caballus, see Horse
Error-catastrophe, *see* Theory
Escherichia coli 24, 96
Euchlanis triquetra 80, 81
Evolution 103
– of ageing 102
– of genes 72
– of genome 24
– of life-span 23, 102
– of viruses 33
Excision-repair 22, 24, 31
Expectation of life 8
see also Life-span

Felis catus, see Cat
Fibroblast cultures 26, 40
– –, age of donor and 27, 28
– –, chicken 40
– –, life-span of 28, 40
– –, man 22, 27, 28, 30, 31, 40
– –, mouse 40
– –, progeria and 22, 30
– –, rat 40
– – time of subculturings 54
– –, tissue of origin and 28
– –, virus and 32–34
– –, von Recklinghausen's syndrome and 41
– –, xeroderma pigmentosum and 22

Finger-ridge count 73
Fission 67, 68, 92
Fitness 2, 12, 46, 80, 102, 103
Flax 72
5-Fluorouracil 30
Fruitfly, *see Drosophila*

Gallus gallus, see Chicken
Gametogenesis 43, 59, 60–75, 89, 91
Gene control 73, 74, 91
– evolution 72
– frequency 9, 46
–, globin 23
–, histone 23
–, major genes and life-span 10, 11
–, minor 12, 52, 65
– mutations 11, 18, 70
– pleiotropy 47, 102
– redundancy 22–24
–, unique 25
Genealogy, *see* Human pedigrees
Genetic basis of ageing 1, 4–19
– control of transformation 39
– equilibrium 47
– homeostasis 47
– redundancy 22–24
– theory of ageing, *see* Theory
Genome evolution 24
Genotype frequency 9
Germ cells, *see* Cell; Gametogenesis
– line 42
Globin genes 23
Goldfinch 14
Growth, ageing and 45–54
–, carrot 41
– cessation 81
– control 38, 89
–, mutations affecting 101
–, parental age and 65
– rate 103
– –, bacteria 96
– –, *Drosophila melanogaster* 51–53
– –, life-span and 45–54, 86, 96, 99
– –, mice 45–48, 99
– –, natural variations of 49, 51
– –, rat 45, 48–50, 99
– –, selection for 46–48, 51, 52
– –, *Tribolium castaneum* 51–53
– retardation 45